How to Stop Colds, Allergies & More

Carole S. Ramke

How to Stop Colds, Allergies & More

http://www.howtostopcolds.com

Printed in the United States of America:
CreateSpace, North Charleston, South Carolina

Paperback First Edition
ISBN: 1-4774-0610-7
ISBN-13: 9781477406106

Library of Congress Control Number: 2012908202

Disclaimer

The purpose of this book is to share health and wellness information gathered over many years of personal research and experience. It is in no way meant to be prescriptive, and it by no means replaces professional medical advice. Readers are responsible for their own choices, actions, and results.

Neither the author nor the publisher accepts responsibility for the accuracy of the information and shall have no liability or responsibility to any person or entity with respect to any loss, damage, or injury caused, or alleged to be caused, directly or indirectly, by the consequences of use or misuse of information contained herein.

References are provided for informational purposes only and do not constitute endorsement of any website, publication, or product. Brand names are used only to enable the reader to compare products, and the author does not own any interest in same.

Dedication

In memory of

Dr. Gerard F. Judd, Ph.D.,

who gave mankind a simple way

to stop colds and allergies

Acknowledgments

Few worthwhile endeavors can be done alone, and I thank my husband for being my closest ally in experimenting with these simple procedures for staying well. His encouragement and support have been invaluable in getting this information published. Thanks also to friends and relatives for experimenting with the methods and giving me their input.

Special thanks go to my friend and fellow Master Gardener, Don Auderer, for the inspiring cover photograph—which to him was just one of many in his artistic photographic gallery. I know it took true grit for him to let me impose my book title and name across his work.

A special thank you also goes to my editor, Susan Redfearn. She worked wonders on my ramblings—but allowed me to do things my way when I insisted, which was often.

Last, I appreciate receiving permission from the following organizations to append their news releases to further describe the latest advances in using nutritional supplements:

Orthomolecular Medicine News Service: Andrew W. Saul, Ph.D., Editor-In-Chief

University of California, San Diego Health Sciences: Kim Edwards, Senior Public Information Officer

Vitamin D Council: John D. Cannell, Ph.D., Founder

Contents

Introduction

If you are tired of having colds and allergies, and if you want to try something that works, this book has been written for you.

This is not a conventional health book, and I am not a health-care professional. I hope the "how-to" title will appeal to anyone who has the motivation to stop a cold without a doctor's intervention. If you do not assume responsibility for your own health, please leave this book on the shelf for someone who is more self-reliant.

The cover is not conventional either, compared to those of other books in this category. I wanted to convey the optimism of better times ahead and the possibility of enjoying nature once again by those who have been restricted by their allergies.

I have provided a summary of remedies as Appendix A, which can be copied for quick reference. There is no implication that the steps should be done in this order, or even that more than one step may be needed at a time.

Significant articles regarding supplements are appended to add to your discovery and understanding. The articles have their own references and sources for further information.

I enjoyed writing the book. I hope you will benefit from reading it and will enjoy relief from colds, allergies, and more for the rest of your life.

Chapter 1
Orientation

Your health is your most valuable possession. Your body is the only home you will ever have in this life, and you should assume full responsibility for the use and care of it. There is no instruction manual. You can either play it by ear and hope for the best, or you can take charge and decide what is right for you.

I am the world's best expert on what works for me. I use first-hand observations, search for second opinions from numerous sources, and use my own judgment as to how to stay healthy and well. I don't want to bore you with stories about myself, but my journey through life provides the background of everything I have learned. So I will share personal experiences to explain observations that may or may not agree with the consensus of public opinion. My hope is that you will use some of this information to improve your health and then share this knowledge with others.

Actually, I never dreamed I would write a book. When taking a seminar last year, I was asked to select a door prize. I picked up a little inspirational book, and before I got home I decided that I should find a way to share my most valuable discoveries with as many people as possible.

Putting my personal experiences into writing is a little scary, because I have always been a very private person. On the other hand, there are important things I have learned that are not being brought into public awareness.

Much of the common knowledge about health and wellness that we embrace today came to us through advertising, as well as government, corporate, and even professional agendas. Most big research projects regarding health are financed by pharmaceutical companies. We think the Food and Drug Administration is taking care of us, but we cannot rely on government agencies to have our best interests at heart.

We are constantly bombarded with information from all directions. Much of it is contradictory and there are many misconceptions that are not being corrected. One would think in this day of advanced technology and communication that this would not be the case—but it is.

For example, new drugs become available which are supposed to be miracle cures. Then they are taken off the market because of some of the side effects—which can actually include stroke and death. We hear negative reports about vitamin E on the evening news, without any mention that only synthetic vitamin E was used in the study. Fluoride is supposed to stop tooth decay and is added to the water supply across the country, although it is a known toxin and there is no minimum daily requirement for it as a supplement. We are told that the only way to feed the world is through genetic engineering. Then we hear about the mysterious demise of the honeybee and the compromise of heirloom seeds. Most people don't even know that almost all of the food available at their supermarket contains at least one unidentified, genetically-modified ingredient. And there is no requirement for labeling in America.

It is said there is no cure for the common cold because it is impossible to develop a vaccine against hundreds of viruses, which may be capable of mutation. We are advised that the best defense is to wash our hands, even though some of the culprits are airborne. This is just a sampling of things we should be concerned about.

I certainly can't solve the problems of the world in one little volume. But thanks to my many years of researching to solve my own problems and to raise healthy children, I have found some effective solutions along the way. They don't involve taking drugs or even using herbs. Some of these remedies involve a different way to use mouthwash or the type of soap to use. All of the solutions are very inexpensive—which I believe will be helpful in today's economy.

There may never be a cure for the common cold. But I have not had a cold, a headache, or a lingering reaction to airborne allergens for almost eight years; and I feel it is my responsibility to tell you what I have discovered.

Who am I?

I have always loved a good hunt—Easter eggs, meteorites, and ancestors, just to name a few.

As a child, I enjoyed studying grammar, math, and science. I didn't much care for history. I would study enough to ace the course and then try to forget everything about the past. I didn't take it seriously when people said we had to understand the past to avoid making the same mistakes in the future. They were right. On the other hand, sometimes we need to turn loose of old sayings and practices that are outdated or proven wrong.

My paternal grandmother was a family historian, having been orphaned at a young age and raised by her grandmother. She loved to tell really old stories—including one about my fifth great-grandfather having been a drummer with George Washington. My generation thought, "Yeah, sure." Then a distant cousin came to visit with my grandmother and brought documentation, including copies of pay vouchers from the National Archives. That woke us up. Valley Forge, huh?

This led to years of historical research in musty libraries from Texas back to Virginia, as well as trips to historical sites up and down the East Coast. In my search for Hubbard Stephens, I learned more about American history than they could ever teach in school. What a great hunt it was. You never knew when some nugget of information would tie in with something else.

Another lesson from genealogy is that it is best to share your information in every way possible. Some researchers want to keep their secrets—after working so hard to find them. But the more I helped others, the more they helped me. And the more I learned, the more different sources tied in with what I knew.

I finally put genealogy on the back burner, when I heard that if you go back twenty generations you may have as many as a million ancestors. That put everything in perspective instantly! It was great fun while it lasted, but I had to admit that there were more important pursuits to occupy my time and attention.

I am at the same kind of crossroad right now. Numerous stories are racing through my mind that might be more fun to talk about. But I really need to share my most valuable health discoveries, so that you can benefit from them too.

My first memory that is relevant to this topic was an experience when I was in the first grade. They still had nap time back then, right after lunch. My teacher would pull down the dark shades and work on a little project to make silhouette cutouts of each child—to give to our parents for Christmas. I remember hearing her apologize to my mother because she had to draw mine with my mouth open. I couldn't breathe with it closed, because I always had a cold or allergies. It also looked as though my eyelashes were at about half-mast. I was not a well child.

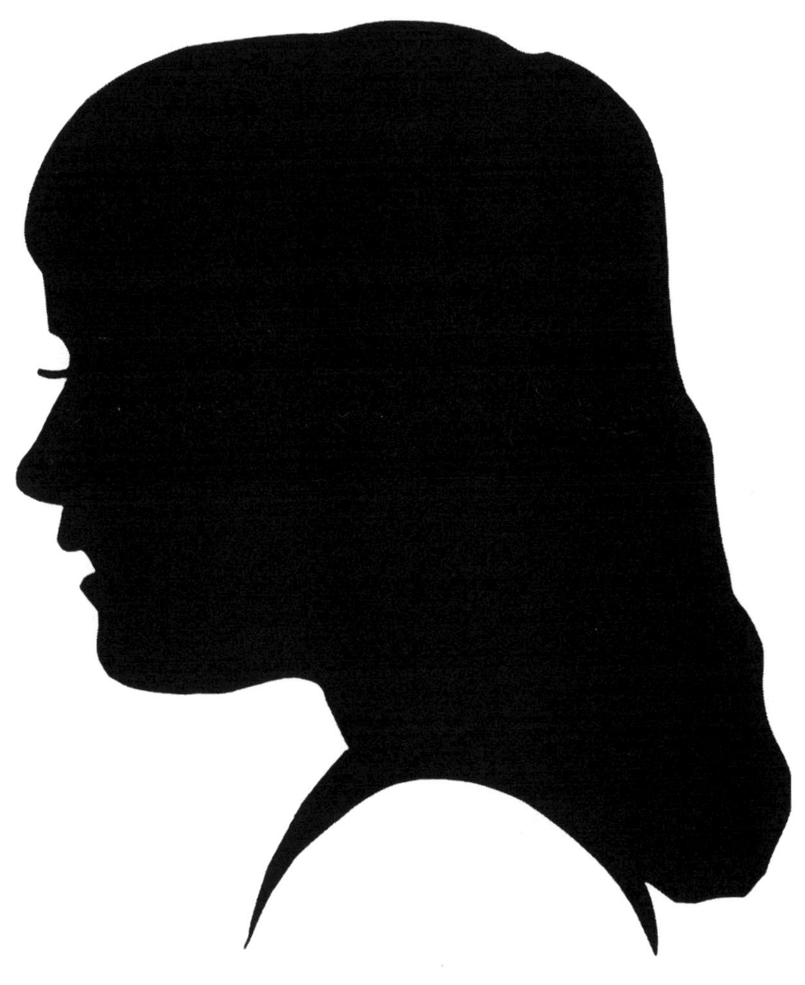

Silhouette of Author, Age 6

Shortly after that, I had my tonsils taken out. I was unconcerned about the whole thing and only looked forward to the ice cream that was promised. What a letdown it was when I couldn't enjoy it. Unfortunately, the procedure didn't end my problems with colds and allergies.

There was something about Christmas that didn't add up either. How could Santa have brought us that heavy electric train and still have had enough room in his sleigh for toys for our whole neighborhood—much less the rest of the world? Okay. Since I was a first child, I had to agree it was in my best interest to pretend to believe. At least my parents always gave valid answers when I asked "Why?" about something. It disturbed me when my friends would get the response, "Because I said so." I assume everyone wants to know where they stand, and there shouldn't be very many situations in life where we have to pretend to believe in Santa.

Years later, when I was planning for college, my mother asked me if I wanted to be a teacher, a secretary, or a nurse. Those were the only options. It was fortunate that I chose secretary because I found that I could get a job in almost any business or profession. I regret not taking chemistry and physiology, but I was too busy taking business courses.

My only exposure to the medical profession was my first job as secretary to an ophthalmologist, while my husband finished his military service. So I am certainly not a doctor, and nothing in this book should be considered medical advice. My subject is just wellness—not medicine.

We had to live very frugally when my husband went back to college, but I was able to put him through architecture school. I learned a lot about architecture and construction along the way, which comes in handy each time we build a house ourselves or tackle various do-it-yourself projects. This has little to do with the subject of this book, other than to say I am serious about doing things myself.

My second job was as secretary in the advertising department of a newspaper. Part of my work was to check the ads in the first edition. I have kept the habit of reading the paper every day since then, but not so much the ads. It is good continuing education to learn everything in the present and keep up with new discoveries and history in the making.

My third job was as secretary to an attorney. I helped with searches of public records. When computer research first became available to law firms, I ran queries for the attorneys, until such time that enough young attorneys could do it themselves. I have worked for law firms ever since, including about 30 years as legal administrator (office manager) for several firms.

I was self-taught. I didn't mind saying, "I don't know, but I'll find out." That pretty much describes my wellness insights also. I enjoy searching for answers and solving problems. The beauty of just searching for the truth is that there is no deadline. Sometimes, if there is no apparent answer, it is better to do nothing, rather than to do something even if it is wrong. The answer might come to me tomorrow.

The Internet is a wonderful resource for learning, if you can weed out the trash. Since I don't have regimented ideas about health topics, I can read all the angles with an open mind and occasionally find an Easter egg peaking out where others have walked right over it.

Did you visualize the egg in black and white or full color? Just curious.

It might seem odd that a chemist found what he said was a cure for the common cold. I tried to tell a doctor about it, and she said she didn't believe in miracle cures! I didn't think it was a miracle. I thought it was common sense. It was so simple—how could you *not* try it and see if it worked?

Most people are almost brainwashed to believe there is no way to avoid the common cold. When I tell them about the protocol devised by a chemist, they look at me with a blank stare. If I see them at the supermarket the next week, they might be comparing prices on cough syrup. I guess we are conditioned to think that colds and allergies are a fact of life, and we just have to put up with them.

I can certainly understand, because that was the way I felt. I was afraid my post-nasal drip would drive people crazy, because I was always coughing. I wondered if it was because of having had my tonsils removed that the drip seemed to go straight into my lungs. I would take medications to try to stop it, but nothing really worked. I felt like Typhoid Mary more often than I care to remember. It is really embarrassing to think of all the years that I went to work stuffed up, half-sick, and brain-dulled from over-the-counter medications. When I wasn't coughing, I was constantly clearing my throat. I hope that everyone I ever worked with will accept my sincere apologies.

My life is different now. The drainage is history, just by using the easy steps outlined in the next chapter. I can't avoid all bacteria, viruses, and allergens, but I can make them irrelevant.

I am reminded of a family story about a favorite niece, when she was about four years old. After going shrimping with friends, my husband had made a big pot of gumbo for the evening meal. In the midst of compliments among the crowd, she suddenly burst into tears, pushed herself back from the table and cried, "I just can't put up with it anymore!" Not realizing that a child's taste buds may be more sensitive than his own, her uncle had been too generous with the Tabasco and other seasonings.

Just imagine how many illnesses and emergency room visits could be avoided if everyone would try these simple suggestions and take responsibility for their own health. My hope is that one or more of the insights in this book will change your life, as they have mine, and that you just won't put up with it anymore!

Chapter 2
The Common Cold

There was an old joke about a man who went to the doctor because he had a cold. He was told to take some pills, but that didn't help. He went back and got a shot, but that didn't help either. On his third visit, the doctor told him to take a bath, open the windows and stand in the draft. The man said, "But doctor, if I do that I might get pneumonia." The doctor replied, "That's true, but I can cure pneumonia!"

The cold virus is the most common infectious disease in the United States; and it is the main reason we visit our physicians, even though there is little they can do for effective treatment. It is said that Americans have over a billion colds per year.

The term *cold*, describing a viral infection of the upper respiratory tract, apparently evolved because it was most common in cold weather. Experts today say that cold weather does not cause us to get sick. Some believe that, since many viruses and bacteria do not survive in higher than normal body temperatures, it is likely that nasal passages chilled by cold weather would be less able to fend them off. During the winter, people are more often in closed spaces with less humidity and air exchange, where they may be exposed to more illnesses. Also, dryness of the throat and nasal membranes may make the surfaces more vulnerable to attack.

The latest speculation on why colds are more frequent in the winter is because we get less sunshine during cold weather. It has been discovered that 85% of Americans are deficient in vitamin D, which is key in boosting immunity.

Everyone who breathes gets germs, dust, and other irritants into their nose and sinuses. The most common advice from the experts is to wash your hands frequently to avoid illness. This is certainly helpful, but it doesn't prevent exposure to airborne bacteria and viruses.

Our saliva contains an enzyme called lysozyme, which kills bacteria that get into our mouth. Disease-causing organisms that are swallowed are said to be killed by digestive juices. However, those that enter the nose, sinuses, and lungs may find shelter—especially if extra congestion is present. The experts are now realizing that when the body overreacts to germs and irritants, the resulting congestion can provide an environment for infections to set in.

Mucus is a clear, lubricating secretion which is normal and beneficial to the membranes in our nose and sinuses. But it becomes prone to infection when it is abundant and thick. So we can't afford to let this happen, if we want to stay well. Coughing is also a normal response to keep our nose and lungs clear and in optimum condition. When we have to cough too much, however, it can lead to hoarseness, pain, and fatigue.

Many of the over-the-counter cold remedies and cough syrups we used in the past have been discontinued because of various side effects—including liver damage. Even if you use those that are still available, they don't really make you feel well or stop a cold. Nasal sprays can be problematic also.

We are beginning to see more alternative recommendations, such as the use of neti pots for cleansing the sinus passages. While this can be an effective way to eliminate congestion, it is an unneeded expense.

Even more alarming than all the unnecessary medications and paraphernalia, surgery is now being performed to enlarge the passages. Oh, my goodness!

I always thought that if germs invaded my nose, it was inevitable that I would be sick for a week or two. Then, more often than not, I would have further complications. But now I know that if I sneeze or get the sniffles, it's not too late to put a stop to it immediately. By keeping my nasal passages and sinuses free of congestion, I can avoid colds, sinus infections, headaches, hay fever, and all kinds of respiratory complications. Too simple, you say? Please bear with me, and you may be pleased with the results.

All you need is a supply of cotton swabs, a mild mouthwash, salt, filtered water, and buffered vitamin C powder. You might want to keep some 3% hydrogen peroxide on hand also. Over-the-counter remedies, antibiotics, and various other prescription drugs can be totally unnecessary—not to mention surgery.

My recommended procedure is as easy as brushing your teeth, yet it is unknown to most people. It was introduced by Gerard F. Judd, Ph.D., in "A Cure for the Common Cold," in the November, 2004, issue of Acres U.S.A., an eco-agriculture publication. Parts of this article are reprinted with permission from Acres U.S.A. (www.acresusa.com).

Over the past eight years, I have made a few modifications to the way I use Dr. Judd's instructions; so I will describe my version here, while giving him full credit for the original version.

Unfortunately, Dr. Judd died in 2007, before I thought about trying to thank him for changing my health and my life.

How did Dr. Judd, a chemist, discover how to stop the common cold? Actually, I don't know if he had a eureka moment or just took advantage of something he had known for a long time. In his article he said:

> Early in my chemistry studies at the University of Utah I learned that when proteins are contacted by alcohol they are denatured, that is, they turn into a different form, which in fact destroys them. For example, when I dripped egg white into alcohol, it turned into a solid. This reaction has something to do with the incompatibility of the alcohol-water-hydroxy groups (OH) and the protein-amide groups (CONH2).
>
> All viruses are protein in nature and have a protein coat. Bacteria are protein in nature. Both of them are destroyed by alcohol (denaturization), and therefore all ailments due to viruses and bacteria are subject to this treatment.

Dr. Judd recommended using a mouthwash with 14% alcohol for several of the steps listed below. I cannot print the brand name of the mouthwash he used. Just be aware that some mouthwashes may be too harsh or contain different percentages of alcohol and various ingredients that may not be suitable for this use. As an alternative, Dr. Judd suggested using vodka, diluted to 14% alcohol. See Appendix B for more information if you choose to dilute vodka or want to consider other alternatives.

Obviously, alcohol is the ingredient that kills germs. This is nothing new. Alcohol has been used for medicinal purposes throughout recorded history, but it seems to be no longer taken seriously other than as an ingredient in cough syrups or hand sanitizers. Even though I don't drink, I find myself in the awkward position of asking you to consider the use of diluted vodka (ethyl alcohol) as a preventative for a surprising number of conditions which affect millions of people.

Here is my version of Dr. Judd's instructions for symptoms related to colds:

Sore Throat

Gargle with mouthwash or diluted vodka (14% alcohol) to put a stop to it quickly.

I remember swabbing my throat with a strong mouthwash as a teenager and trying not to gag. It did stop the sore throat, but the infection would always go into my nose anyway. The next step is a simple prevention for that.

Sneezing, Coughing, Nasal Congestion, Sinus Drip

Dip a cotton swab in 14% alcohol and run it up the nostrils to stop viruses, bacteria, and even the histamine reaction. Be gentle, please.

I call this the "nip-it trick." Coating the nasal passages with a mild alcohol wash is really the key to preventing colds, because you can kill viruses and bacteria in an area that we normally ignore. This also shuts down the overreaction of histamine to any airborne irritants. You don't need to do it on a daily basis, but only if you get the sniffles or feel like you may be coming down with something. It is very quick and easy, and you will be amazed how fast the symptoms disappear.

I don't think you have to do it immediately for it to work. But I never waste time because I don't want to be bothered with congestion or sneezing any longer than necessary. It is also useful if you wake up on a winter morning and your nose is dry from the heating system running all night.

Some people are shocked at the idea of using anything containing alcohol in their nose. A friend told me her doctor said not to do that because alcohol is too drying. To the contrary, Dr. Judd said:

> Since alcohol is a very good wetting agent (its surface tension is 40 dynes, compared to water at 92 and a soap solution at 52), it will remove all materials from the surface, including pollens and even the histamine allergen which the body makes.

So water would apparently be more drying to the nose than alcohol. He went on to say:

> Alcohol is an excellent wetter, breaking up water from its large structures down into tiny, perhaps even molecular sizes. These tiny structures get closer to the surface, facilitating their removal.

He was referring to clearing any congestion that clings to the membranes in the nose.

Other people have commented that alcohol does not kill all germs. I have found that we don't need to exterminate all microbes but just set them back a little, if they are invading our nose or lungs, so our body's own defenses can stay in control.

The nip-it trick reminds me of Don Knotts (as Barney) saying, "Nip it in the bud." Most of the time, this is all you need to do to stay well.

Watering or Irritated Eyes

Dr. Judd recommended further diluting the 14% alcohol with 15 parts of water for an eye wash to clean pollens, allergens, and histamine from the eyes, as well as destroying bacteria and viruses that might be present. This would make a solution of 1% alcohol or slightly less. I have tried it, and it worked very well—even when I had redness like pink eye (conjunctivitis). If this simple remedy did not work quickly, or if there was any possibility of a foreign particle in the eye, I would, of course, see an ophthalmologist.

I have found that a weaker solution is effective also. Sometimes I just put one drop of 14% alcohol into a little eye cup and fill it with filtered water or saline. This is much more diluted, but it works great if I feel like I have a bit of lint in my eye or any minor irritation. My doctor said he had no objections.

Infection Spreading Into the Lungs

Heat four teaspoons of 14% alcohol just until steam starts coming up. Inhaling the vapor will destroy the germs trying to invade your lungs.

Dr. Judd wrote:

> Boiling four teaspoons of [mouthwash or vodka diluted to 14%] on the stove permits alcohol vapor to come off at a warm temperature of about 55 C. Inhaling one or two dozen breaths of this vapor kills all bacteria and viruses in the lungs. One volume of liquid gives only .00005 volume of vapor. This treatment ended a cold in my lungs for the first time in many years.
>
> I believe this treatment could mean the end of the common cold, viral pneumonia, bronchial pneumonia, Ebola, and other viral and bacterial diseases, because they are all proteins in nature.

I thought the procedure sounded comforting enough, since such a small amount of alcohol would be entering my lungs; but I was confused about how to boil only four teaspoons of liquid. When the day came that I had to try this, because germs had gotten past my nose and throat, I found a simple solution. I measured four teaspoons of 14% alcohol into a stainless steel measuring cup and heated it just until vapor started appearing. Then I could turn off the burner and carry the cup to a safer spot to inhale the steam and destroy the germs trying to invade my lungs. It provided instant relief.

If you don't have a stainless steel measuring cup, a ceramic or stainless steel pot could be heated enough on one side to start the evaporation. I suppose you could warm the four teaspoons of whatever nasal wash (14% alcohol) you are using in a microwave, but I would be concerned about microwaving such a small quantity of anything and the danger that it could dry up or just burn off the alcohol too fast and make the treatment ineffective. I really don't think microwaving would be a good idea.

Being able to stop an infection that is spreading into my lungs has been beyond incredible for me. The delicate alcohol vapor coats the surfaces being infected and stops the irritation so effectively that it is hard to believe—unless you experience it for yourself.

I think this step does need to be done as soon as you feel an infection invading your lungs. It might still help later. But as congested and painful as my lungs used to get from coughing, it is hard to imagine that a tiny amount of vapor could work at that point. For the past eight years, I have had no congestion in my lungs; so I can't speak from experience, because I have not had occasion to try it at that stage. I guess you could do it more than once over a period of time, but I wouldn't use more than four teaspoons at once. More research is needed.

Clearing the Head

Inhale heated salt water from the hand to the nose, so that mucus is dissolved and removed from the nose, throat, sinuses, and back to the Eustachian tubes—until the head is cleared. Then use the first two steps above, if needed, for complete removal.

Clearing mucus from your head is the key to getting rid of a cold that sets in before you can do the nip-it trick. It can only work if you try it. I seldom have to do this, but it has never failed to work for me. That's a pretty good record.

Add a level one-half teaspoon of plain salt to a cup (8 oz.) of filtered or distilled hot water. Stir to dissolve and make it isotonic. Wash your hands thoroughly. Bend over a sink and inhale the solution from your hand into your nose. Be careful that it is not too hot; but the warmer the solution, the more the mucus is dissolved and removed from tissue surfaces and can be spit out. Mucus can be removed from the mouth, nose, throat, sinuses, and clear back to the Eustachian tubes as described by Dr. Judd. Eliminating the congestion significantly reduces the risk of complications, by giving the infection no place to lodge.

Using salt water is, of course, an old-time remedy; but any time I tried sniffing salt water in the past, I felt like I was going to drown. I think the key to success is sniffing the salt water from your hand and keeping your mouth open. That limits the amount of water you can inhale; and, by necessity, you are bending way over the sink to do it. Anyway, when I do it Dr. Judd's way, I am in no danger of drowning at all.

The second point is that the water should be as warm as you can tolerate it, without being too hot. The warmer it is, the more germs it can kill. If the water is too cool, it defeats your purpose by causing tissues to swell. Your head really can be cleared. Just be sure your hands are clean before you start.

Dr. Judd did not specify any particular type of salt. It seemed to me that iodized salt was less comfortable than regular salt. But I believe all table salts contain anti-caking agents to keep them flowing freely. Some sources of information about nasal washing recommend using sea salt. Others recommend using canning and pickling salt because it is free of any added conditioners. Kosher salt should be good also.

Salt in the proper ratio and without any additives should not burn at all. Professional divers are trained to take off their goggles and open their eyes in the ocean. Our body and tears contain a large percentage of salt, which is said to be in almost the same ratio as sea water.

There is no need to be stingy with the amount of salt water solution. A cup is enough for me; but you might want to use one level teaspoon of salt and two cups of water—especially if your sinuses are really clogged up. Just take your time and blow it out gently, even if you have to rewarm the salt water.

I have always found it confusing when people specify a glass of water, whether talking about how much water to use in a solution like this or recommending how much water we should drink per day. Glasses come in many sizes. If they are thinking about a juice glass and I am visualizing an iced tea glass, there could be a real misunderstanding. So, in my version of Dr. Judd's instructions,

I use a half teaspoon of salt for each 8 oz. of water, which matches numerous recommendations found on the Internet.

If there is any question about the safety of your water supply, you should use reverse osmosis filtered water, distilled water, or boil your water first and let it cool to a temperature that is very warm but comfortable.

I know this technique sounds like a real chore if you are not familiar with nasal irrigation. I readily admit it is my least favorite tip for staying well. Fortunately, I have only had to resort to this several times in the past eight years; but it is really effective if all else has failed. It truly is not as unpleasant as a cold or a sinus infection.

You should be able to mostly avoid nose blowing, which can send infection to ears and sinus passages and increase swelling and irritation. You might also be able to avoid breathing through your mouth, which has numerous negative effects.

Enhancing Immunity

After using any or all of the above steps that are needed to remove congestion, you should finish up with supplements to boost your ability to fight off any remaining threat. Dr. Judd wrote:

> Extensive research and documentation proves that vitamin C—4,000 milligrams per day—dramatically increases the immune system, which then reduces one's susceptibility to viruses and bacteria. It is best to add 4,000 mg (1 level teaspoon) of ascorbic acid (vitamin C) to a glass with half a teaspoon of baking soda, then add 1 inch of water, let fizz, add more water, and drink.
>
> The sodium ascorbate formed is about 1,000 times more soluble than typical vitamin C pills and far more reactive in increasing immunity.

I agree, and I do not hesitate to take more than that if I feel I might be coming down with something. One teaspoon is usually enough, but on a short-term basis to get over a real threat of illness, I might take several level teaspoons during the day or a half-teaspoon every few hours. I have never had any problems with it. Tablets are not as effective as the powder. They don't dissolve as rapidly, and they all contain fillers. Even if your tablets are 500 mg, you would have to take eight of them to equal 4000 mg.

For convenience, I buy already-buffered Vitamin C (sodium ascorbate) at a health food store, rather than mixing baking soda with ascorbic acid. It is handy to use in juice, smoothies, or plain water any time I want to enhance immunity. The sodium ascorbate powder that I use contains 3380 mg of Vitamin C and 420 mg of sodium per level teaspoon. If you want to avoid the sodium that comes with the bicarbonate of soda used as a buffer, you could use plain ascorbic acid powder and a little sugar or honey with more water or juice to make it palatable, since the ascorbic acid is really sour by itself. My research shows that the sodium in sodium ascorbate is from baking soda and is not the sodium chloride as in table salt, which many doctors recommend avoiding. That is something which would have to be determined by you.

Some sources recommend against taking high doses of vitamin C on a daily basis because it might increase the body's dependence on it. In researching vitamin C, I found that this is highly unlikely, if not impossible. Other sources say you can safely take massive amounts per day to fight various kinds of illnesses. I know it can certainly boost your immunity when needed, so I agree with the latter opinion.

Since it is water soluble, there is no danger of overdosing. When you are fighting illness, you need much more than when you are well. Your body will tell you if you have consumed more than you can absorb, by threatening diarrhea. That is your cue to decrease and level off the dosage until you are well. Chapter 6 and a number of appended articles will provide more detail.

Dr. Judd also recommended a good multivitamin to enhance immunity. I keep trying different formulations, depending on what I think I need. I don't think it is possible to get a good quality multivitamin—with even minimum daily requirements—into one tablet per day. Because of the new discoveries about vitamin D in recent years, I also recommend that you take extra vitamin D3.

That's it! I know it's hard to believe, but these simple procedures can stop the common cold, which will in turn prevent bronchitis, sinus infections, pneumonia, and more. I don't worry any longer about being around coughing people at the grocery store or other crowded places. I don't worry about being exposed to small children with colds. I don't even bother with antibacterial soaps or hand cleaners. I just use plain bar soap.

I enjoy sharing these tips because they work for me—no more headaches, colds, sinus infections, allergy sniffles, chronic coughs, etc. If you will invest in the suggested supplies, you may find, as I did, that all of your over-the-counter medications have expired! Sniffing hot salt water is not fun, but it works. And it's much less expensive than the alternatives.

How to protect children from colds was not addressed by Dr. Judd. The labels on some mouthwashes specify that they should not be used by children under six years old and only with supervision up to age twelve. I agree. A modified version of the nip-it trick which can be used for children will be covered in Chapter 3.

Years ago, a health newsletter recommended using hydrogen peroxide for an earache. Later, I got a pain in my ear and found that I had somehow lost or misfiled the article. So I poured a few drops of 3% hydrogen peroxide into my ear and waited a few minutes. The bubbling noise was soothing and the pain went away. I didn't remember if the article had stated whether this could be used for children. Then another special niece, who is a pediatric nurse, came to visit. I mentioned my question to her and she said they use this for children in hospital wards all the time!

So to my version of the protocol devised by Dr. Judd, I should add:

Earache

Pour several drops of 3% hydrogen peroxide into the ear and let it bubble for a few minutes. Then drain. Dry the outer ear. You can clean the large part of the ear canal with a cotton swab, but don't probe toward the inner ear. Just leave it moist.

I have read from other sources that just putting 3% hydrogen peroxide into each ear for a few minutes can stop colds and sore throats in addition to earaches. It can be used more than once in each ear until no more bubbling is heard. So this might be a solution for very young children as well as for anyone who wants to avoid using alcohol for preventing colds.

An acquaintance told me that her mother would put 3% peroxide in her ear when she was young. But the bubbling noise scared her so badly that she would sit up and drain it out before it could do any good. It might be worthwhile to introduce a child to the bubbling effect on a wound or to talk about how it will sound before using it in their ear. Maybe you could come up with other ideas to make children more receptive to the experience. Also, take care not to get it into their eyes.

Dry air caused by winter heating systems can be a problem, especially for children. Humidifiers can be helpful, but they can be problematic if not strictly maintained. One solution is geothermal heating, which is more gentle and comfortable. The downside is that this type of system is more expensive and can be difficult to install, other than in new construction. The initial investment, however, can be offset by savings in monthly electric bills.

Wikipedia says, "Due to lack of studies, it is not currently known whether increased fluid intake improves symptoms or shortens respiratory illness, and a similar lack of data exists for the use of heated humidified air." Since learning the nip-it trick, I have not needed to be concerned about humidity at all.

Many old remedies for fighting the common cold involved sipping hot tea or eating chicken soup, etc. This old wives' tale was found to be true. Chicken contains cysteine, which can thin the mucus in your lungs. I like chicken soup and continue to enjoy it occasionally, even though I no longer have colds. If you don't like chicken soup, however, you may never have to eat it again, thanks to Dr. Judd. You should not have congestion in your lungs if you follow his advice.

What about the old question of whether to feed a cold and starve a fever? Although it is okay for a person with a common cold and little or no fever to eat normal meals, a recent study found that a person with viral influenza would benefit from light broths and purified water, while their liver is working on both digestion and detoxification at the same time. This is just one more problem that might be avoided by a preemptive strike with a nip-it trick. I'm laughing, but very serious!

If you are a hypochondriac, these simple techniques may not be for you. The grandmother I mentioned earlier enjoyed going to various doctors without telling them what was being prescribed by others. She was actually taking medications to fight the side effects of other medications. She loved going to the hospital for tests about once a year. My dad said she had claimed to have cancer ever since she found out there *was* such a thing. Finally a perceptive doctor requested that all old medication be removed from her home and told her that if she didn't get well enough to go home, he would have to put her into a nursing home. She checked out that very day and was still gardening in her mid-nineties!

Some people just can't handle change. When I worked for an eye doctor many years ago, he told the story of how he was able to restore the sight of a young woman who was legally blind. It brought tears to my eyes twice—once on hearing about how she was able to see again, and the second time on learning that she had committed suicide when she discovered that her disability checks would be discontinued.

Yes, these are extreme examples; but I want you to realize that you might experience a new paradigm. You will be exposed to just as many colds and the same allergens, but you can stop all adverse reactions—if you have the determination to stock the few supplies and use them according to directions. There is no magic pill, but none are needed. You will never know if it works, unless you do it yourself.

We really don't need a cure for the common cold. The typical symptoms are caused by the body's immune response to viral infections, rather than to any actual tissue destruction by the viruses. You can stop the reactions and make the symptoms go away. Don't waste time nursing symptoms.

Here is a very brief summary of the strategy for stopping colds:

- If your throat starts getting sore, gargle with 14% alcohol.
- For sneezing, coughing, congestion, or nasal drip, use the nip-it trick.
- For watering or irritated eyes, use an eye cup with an extremely mild alcohol solution.
- For infection spreading into the lungs, inhale the vapor from only four teaspoons of 14% alcohol.
- To clear the head of congestion, inhale very warm salt water from hand to nose and blow out gently.
- To enhance immunity, use powdered vitamin C, multivitamins, and vitamin D3.
- For an earache, use several drops of 3% hydrogen peroxide, let it bubble, and then drain.

It is up to you to notice when a symptom is beginning and take the appropriate action. At the first sign of a cold, try the nip-it trick. Once is usually enough. If you should wake up with a sinus infection, complete with fever, you might have to use almost all of the procedures, but I have found that it is possible to overcome it in one day!

Various estimates of the economic impact of loss of work and medical expenses of the common cold in America each year are astounding. Thinking back on all the colds and allergic reactions that I alone experienced during my working years, the total misery and loss of productivity nationwide must be beyond comprehension.

If everyone could use these simple techniques to avoid colds, along with the resulting complications and secondary infections, just imagine the difference in economic impact, the use of medical resources for more important needs, and the improvement in quality of life for all.

Chapter 3
Stop Reactions to Airborne Allergens

The headline of Dr. Judd's article did not point out that he had a remedy for allergies. Maybe he was not bothered by allergies. He just referred to being able to remove histamine allergens. When I saw those words in his little article, it was like a revelation from heaven, because I realized the potential significance for me.

Apparently I have always been sensitive to airborne allergens—such as pollens, perfume, smoke, and dust. As a youngster, I knew that sweeping the garage would give me a headache. I never thought of it as an allergy. I just knew it wasn't good to breathe a lot of dirt. My mother probably thought my protest at being assigned that chore was because I preferred more pleasant pastimes. I can't deny that, but I wasn't hopelessly lazy. I would volunteer to vacuum the whole house, if my sister would only agree to clean the bathroom. A little negotiation was allowed, as long as we got everything done.

Thinking back, I believe my dad must have had the same problems with breathing dust as I have. He always insisted that we should not flip the broom up, when sweeping, and pointed out how the dust took to the air, when observed in sunlight in his shop doorway.

I guess everything is a matter of degree. I never noticed any reaction to vacuuming, while some people say they can't tolerate the microscopic particles which that activity can put into the air. In those days, of course, we didn't have micron filters.

I do remember being bothered by heavy perfumes at church. When I was old enough to use some myself, I thought it would be okay. But no—I had to rush home and wash it off because it was making me nauseous.

Pollens didn't seem to bother me, or I wasn't aware of it if they did. We always grew lots of flowers, and my mother made arrangements with them. It wasn't until I was managing an office where a nice bouquet was delivered that I noticed a reaction to some kind of lily. But it wasn't just me. People seemed to be coming out of the woodwork, complaining about the scent. We solved the problem by taking the biggest lily outdoors. We weren't affected by the rest of the flowers. It turned out that the Stargazer lily is notorious for causing allergies, while Asiatic lilies are not as likely to cause a problem.

I know you don't care about the details of what causes my allergies, but these are a few examples of how allergic reactions can wreak havoc with your health—whether you are aware of the causes or not.

If nothing else, please let this be a gentle reminder of problems that others may be experiencing. People who are very sensitive to pet dander, for example, are frequently viewed with disdain by animal lovers, who cannot relate to their very real discomfort.

Headaches

I used to think that I had sinus headaches. For many years I was too often taking antihistamines, which helped a little but caused other symptoms. I finally consulted an ear, nose, and throat specialist, who explained that there was nothing wrong with my sinuses. Instead, the above-mentioned irritants were causing spasms in my sinus and nasal passages—sometimes as long as twelve hours after exposure. I had no idea that being exposed to a smoker, for example, could bother me that much later. The doctor recommended something like ibuprofen for relief, rather than antihistamines. This was an improvement and increased my understanding, but I still had frequent headaches, which could only be relieved by medication.

One of the worst allergy headaches I ever had was after searching for ancestors in the historical library of Duke University. The findings were fantastic; but the musty, yellowed books were my nemesis. Please skip the rest of this paragraph if you have a weak stomach. Okay. I had no ibuprofen to relax the spasms and found myself throwing up on the side of the road on the way home. I don't know if you have ever experienced that kind of sick headache; but after each of the few times such a thing happened to me, I found that the headache disappeared. I wondered if that was the body's way of clearing out the nostrils and letting stomach acid put a stop to the reaction. Anyway, it was quite an indignity to suffer by someone who doesn't even drink. My addiction was genealogy, of course, not alcohol. Little did I know that a slight drop of diluted alcohol actually could have been the solution.

Now I am able to stop allergy headaches immediately, thanks to Dr. Judd. The nip-it trick is a real breakthrough against allergens and histamine reactions. It is just the ticket when you have been exposed to dust, mold, pollens, smoke, perfumes, pet dander, or anything else which can cause congestion or an allergic headache.

When I feel as though I might be having a slight reaction to something, I use a variation of the nip-it trick. Rather than just coating my nostrils, I put a moistened swab into each side of my nose and sniff just a little. This takes the solution into the area of the upper nose and sinuses where the allergic spasms begin. The mild alcohol wash is able to stop the histamine reaction to pollens or whatever the irritant happens to be. It is as simple as that. You can't always get away from irritants, but you can stop the reaction.

Now I don't use any headache medications at all—over-the-counter or otherwise.

I have seen articles recently which speculate that other types of headaches—including migraines—could possibly be triggered by allergies. I have no insight on this, other than the thought that you might want to experiment with this simple remedy and share any discoveries.

Respiratory Allergies

All of the procedures in Chapter 2—including cleaning the eyes—work for allergy problems as well as colds. Even if you don't seem to have any allergies at all, some of the information covered in this chapter will probably benefit you anyway, if only to assist family or friends.

In late December of last year, my husband and I went shopping in another city. On the way home, I noticed that my nose was getting stuffy. Since I was driving, I asked him to hand me a moistened swab. I wouldn't think of dialing my cell phone while driving, because I don't have speed dial or hands-free features. But I didn't need to take my eyes off the road to sniff a little diluted alcohol into each nostril. Before we arrived home about 30 minutes later, the congestion was history.

When we watched the local news that night, we learned that there was a very high level of cedar pollen in the air, which was earlier than usual in our area—probably due to the drought. I never considered myself as being allergic to cedar pollen, although I have heard many people say they do have problems with it. But I can just shrug it off because, as you can see, it is really not a significant problem for me now.

That was the total treatment for an allergic reaction—no tissue, no drugs, no misery. A tiny bit of alcohol stopped the overproduction of histamine in response to an unknown irritant. It seems too simple to be true; but even though the irritant is still in the air, just stopping the trigger somehow stops the overreaction to it.

In my past life, before discovering Dr. Judd's advice, it would have been just a matter of time before I was at my doctor's office, hoping to get antibiotics for some secondary infection. In the meantime, I would have spent many hours blowing my nose, sneezing, taking medications, and coughing until my ribs hurt—not to mention other repercussions like not getting good rest and exercise, having a poor appetite, and being unable to do justice to my family and career obligations.

This simple method for stopping allergic headaches or congestion is effective, no matter whether you know the cause or not. It is not a miracle cure, but rather a mechanical way to help your body avoid sending the hook and ladder trucks to take care of a smoldering candle.

A friend asked me how often I have to use the nip-it trick to avoid reactions to pollens that may be constantly in the air during certain seasons. I guess she thought I would have to walk around with a cotton swab in my hand. Surprisingly, my answer was, "Not very often." For some reason, a histamine reaction seems to perpetuate itself. But when I nip it in the bud, it just gives up and goes away. Somehow, stopping the trigger can enable the body to relax and ignore the irritant.

I never have to treat watering eyes either. My nose is always clear, and my tear ducts are open and can function properly.

My husband discovered that he no longer has to sleep with his mouth open, because he is never congested. I am pleased that he doesn't snore noticeably any more. I wonder if these simple procedures might even help reduce the incidence of sleep apnea, by eliminating (or at least reducing) swelling in the throat, nose, and sinus passages.

Odor Neutralizer

For someone like me, most air fresheners are worse than the odors they are supposed to mask! I discovered an odor neutralizer last year, however, which I can recommend without hesitation. It is made from natural plant oils; and rather than hiding an odor, it eliminates it and leaves no scent of its own after a few seconds. I put it to the acid test.

We had placed an ad in the paper to sell an old car that we weren't driving any more. In the meantime, a predator had killed one of our laying hens. My husband had bagged up the carcass and put it on the back floor of the car to take to the garbage can as he drove past the mailbox. He forgot it was there!

On the first day the ad appeared, I went out to be sure the car was ready to show. Oh Nooooo! I thought we would have to cancel the ad and junk the car. I got on the Internet and found a product called X-O Odor Neutralizer, made in Texas, which was said to remove animal odors naturally, rather than masking them. I drove about 50 miles to get a small bottle of it.

The first person who looked at the car stuck his head through the open window and commented that it was really clean! After a quick test drive, he said he would meet me at the title office. No kidding!

When I am in a small office that gets contaminated with a guest's heavy perfume, this product can erase it from the air. What a relief. The only problem is trying to hold my breath until the visitor leaves! If they don't leave quickly enough, I can always resort to the nip-it trick later.

Suggestions for Children

I had wondered how children could be treated safely with Dr. Judd's methods for stopping the common cold. You don't want them to play with cotton swabs. You don't want them to swallow any mouthwash. I wouldn't want to try to teach them to sniff salt water.

Then last year one of our granddaughters came to stay with us for a few days. She was only six years old. On the first morning she woke up with a runny nose. While she was getting dressed, I sat there sipping my tea and trying to figure out how to help her.

I finally considered my variation of the nip-it trick. I don't have to swab my nostrils thoroughly. Instead, I can put a moistened swab in each side of my nose and sniff slightly until I can taste the mouthwash in my throat. This coats more area than I can reach, and it really goes where it is needed to stop an allergic reaction. There is no danger of drawing it into my lungs because there is not more than half of a drop clinging to the swab.

When my granddaughter came back into the room, I asked her to blow her nose gently with a tissue. Then I handed her a moistened swab and asked her to put it into each side of her nose and sniff just until she could taste the flavor. She looked puzzled but was curious enough about the flavor idea to try it. That seemed to work okay. Then we got busy making blueberry pancakes and forgot about it.

I don't know whether her runny nose had been caused by an allergy or a cold; but it really didn't matter, because her nose was clear for the rest of her visit.

Be Prepared

The most common problem I hear, when I get feedback from friends and relatives, is that when they started feeling a cold or allergy coming on they didn't have the supplies on hand. They had not been able to find a suitable monthwash or powdered vitamin C at Wal-Mart. In our area, we can find powdered ascorbic acid or sodium ascorbate at health food stores. A large bottle of mouthwash with 14% alcohol can be found at most drug stores, or you can see Appendix B for other options.

Don't do as I did and substitute a mouthwash that is entirely too strong, because I had not located any 14% alcohol mouthwash before the first time I needed it. Fortunately, I didn't give up on the procedure after my initial mistake, but went on to try all of the steps correctly—much to my benefit.

The second most common problem was that friends couldn't find my typed directions when needed. So I am including a brief checklist of directions as "Appendix A.1" I recommend that you put a copy in your medicine cabinet along with your supplies. Then you will be prepared to defend yourself when the time comes.

There is another possible use for your medicine cabinet copy of the checklist, especially for senior citizens. If you loan this book to a friend or relative, you could jot down the name of the last person who borrowed it. Then, if you have to stage a recall, you will know where to start. ;-)

Avoid Medications

What is a histamine reaction anyway? Numerous sources say that histamine is part of the body's natural defense system against allergens. When an allergen is detected, the body produces antibodies, mast cells, white blood cells, proteins, and histamines. The response to airborne irritants may include sneezing, watery eyes, and congestion. The over-production of mucus sets up conditions for secondary infections to become established.

The most common treatment advice is to take an antihistamine, which stops the mast cells from producing so much histamine. In my opinion, that is a whole-body treatment to stop a very small localized reaction.

The beauty of Dr. Judd's method is that you can stop the reaction to an airborne allergen right at the source—inside your nose—rather than ingesting medication which can inhibit your ability to think clearly and create other side effects that make you feel miserable. In addition, you can actually get accustomed to not being congested any more. I never dreamed this would be possible.

Perhaps medical research professionals, with much more resources and knowledge than I, can discover why or how these simple techniques prevent colds and allergies. It is more than likely that none will try, however, because there is no money to be made for proving a simple truth. It is much more likely that studies would be done to discredit Dr. Judd's explanation or to find some danger in using common hygiene items and supplements to avoid illness.

I have not been cured of any allergies. I avoid airborne irritants when I can, but I don't have any feeling of panic or stress when I cannot. I enjoy the wonderful gift of knowing how to stop excessive histamine reactions.

Please pay it forward.

Chapter 4
Transdermal Remedies

Don't underestimate what can be absorbed through your skin.

I have read that if you step on a slice of fresh garlic with your bare foot, you will be surprised how fast you can taste it. This is on my list of things to do—if I ever get around to it. In the meantime, I wouldn't be surprised if it is true.

Abscessed Tooth

After discovering Dr. Judd's article on the common cold, I found something he had written about care of the teeth, in which he advised that you could take a swig of mouthwash with 14% alcohol and hold it around an abscessed tooth for five minutes to stop the infection.

I didn't have occasion to use this tip until last year. I had to do it more than once, but it worked. Apparently enough diluted alcohol can be absorbed through the gums in that length of time to kill the infection.

That's more than a little cheaper than a root canal! I don't have proof that there is no sign of an abscess under the tooth, but neither do I know how much infection may be going into my blood stream from old root canals. I can only say that there has been no further hint of infection around that tooth.

Transdermal Observations

After the above-described experience, I started discovering various ways to use common household products that involved absorption through the skin. I had seen the word *transdermal* somewhere, but didn't really grasp the obvious meaning: *through the skin*. In medical dictionaries the term refers to medications administered by patch.

As a child, I remember being shocked by the death of a family friend because he had used some kind of solvent without gloves. That impressed on me the need to avoid bodily contact with harsh chemicals. I guess that was the beginning of my attitude about avoiding contact with various other products containing ingredients that I do not trust. My husband used to think I was overreacting when I would caution him about using commercial products, without adequate protection, while he was rebuilding a car or restoring old boats.

When I started checking into the many ingredients in personal products sold for use on the skin, I was shocked at how many questionable substances are allowed. There is little or no regulation on those products, since they are not to be eaten. That doesn't mean we don't need to be careful.

Substances that are swallowed are thought to be broken down by the digestive process, and we hope any toxins are rejected by the body. But substances that are absorbed through the skin can get into the blood stream and may be distributed to the brain or other organs, before being processed or screened by the liver or kidneys, etc.

I think people are becoming more concerned about exposure to numerous ingredients that we cannot pronounce or understand. Many so-called "green" products are becoming available, but some of them are made to appear safer than they really are.

I used to avoid products with fragrances because of the possibility that I might be allergic to a perfume. Now I know that there is an even more important reason to avoid fragrances. That is because they are allowed to be secret formulas for competition purposes, and manufacturers do not have to list even more dangerous chemicals that may be used.

Several of my friends use organic coconut oil as a skin moisturizer. They say it also makes an excellent conditioner—for use before washing your hair. It can even be used to prevent tangling after shampooing, if you are very careful not to use too much. I was hesitant to try it at first, because it looks like a solid fat. But then I learned that it melts at about 76 degrees and is very smooth and thin. So you can't tell if you like it until you try it.

I try to find items with natural ingredients and try to avoid petroleum products, known carcinogens, etc. Anything claimed to be natural does not have to be safe, however; and even products claimed to be organic do not have to be 100% organic. Some mostly organic products still contain various parabens as preservatives. Parabens are said to be safe by at least one government agency. However, I read that parabens are commonly found in tumors; so it is up to each individual to decide if he or she wants to be exposed to them. There are numerous other examples of questionable ingredients in shampoo, toothpaste, cleaning products, etc.

On the other hand, transdermal absorption can have some interesting beneficial uses. After overcoming my abscessed tooth, I discovered several other ideas I would like to share.

Insect Bites

I know you can soak a small amount of cotton with alcohol and apply it to a bug bite to get good results. This allows more alcohol to soak into the swollen spot than if you just splash it on. I am not using the alcohol to stop an infection, but to reduce a histamine reaction.

My granddaughter lives in an area without mosquitoes. But when she visits with us, they seem to seek her out. When they find her, they cause a big allergic reaction. She loves to use my desktop tape dispenser. So I dampen a wisp of cotton with mouthwash and put it on the bump, then she tears off enough tape to reach past the dampness. This is cheaper than bandage tape and removal is less painful. Then she is not tempted to scratch the spot and turn a minor nuisance into an infection.

Fire ants are common in our area. They can leave a pustule which might stay red and itch for days. I have found that alcohol, allowed to soak in from a bit of cotton, can eliminate the pus and itch, although the spot may still remain red for some time.

Skin Fungus (Tinea Versicolor)

Baking soda, sprinkled on a rash on my husband's back, had no noticeable benefit. However, mixing it with almost hot water and soaking it into a soft cotton cloth, which was then placed on the skin for minutes at a time, gave an entirely different result.

Tinea versicolor is caused by a fungus, which is said not to be contagious because it is normally on everyone's skin. Apparently, it is not known why some people have a reaction to it or their body chemistry lets it get out of control. But it is unsightly and it sometimes itches.

My husband has had spots on his back since he was a teenager. He thought he was allergic to sunshine. It was later diagnosed as tinea versicolor. A dermatologist prescribed some pills. He warned that the medication was only to be taken for short periods at a time, because it could kill the patient along with the fungus causing the rash. Even after putting up with side effects and feeling foolish for taking a poison, my husband didn't experience much relief.

Then a liquid was prescribed, which I had to rub on his back. I didn't appreciate having the skin peel off my hand, especially since the remedy failed to cure his rash. Later, we tried powdering his back with corn starch, which is commonly used for diaper rash. That helped a little in hot weather but didn't get his condition under control.

Next, we tried powdering with baking soda, since I knew it was used as an antifungal remedy in organic gardening. It didn't work very well either. Then I decided to make use of the concept of liquid absorption into the skin. We made a slurry of baking soda in warm water and plastered his back. The next morning we found the spots had virtually disappeared!

This was a miraculous remedy for something that had been a nuisance for many years. It still isn't 100% cured, but now he can easily keep the condition to a minimum and stay comfortable.

The only problem we had with our treatment was that it was messy. The baking soda gets crusty as it dries, and the poor person can get chilled while trying to let the solution soak in.

The next time, we tried making a much thinner mixture, using about a tablespoon of baking soda to each cup of water. We warmed it on the stove and used a piece of soft cotton cloth to apply to each area for a few minutes. Then we could rewarm the water as needed to soak the cloth each time it cooled off. It wasn't necessary to make the solution so thick, but to let the solution soak in well.

I think a teaspoon of baking soda for each cup of water may be strong enough; but my husband likes to make it stronger, just to be sure it is effective. You might want to experiment to see what strength works best for you. The recipe used by organic gardeners is four teaspoons to a gallon of water for spraying fungal diseases on plants, so even that strength may be enough, if allowed to soak into the skin.

I don't know if baking soda works just because it is alkaline or because it has other properties that kill fungus. But who cares? It is my opinion that strong anti-fungal medications are not needed for use on tinea versicolor.

Right after the last time we treated his rash, my husband complained that it was itching more than usual. I did an Internet search for "anti-fungal foods." There on the first page I saw something I already had on hand—coconut oil. I learned that it contains caprylic acid, a medium chain saturated fatty acid, which can inhibit fungal growth, topically as well as internally. My hands felt a little dry after helping him with the baking soda solution, so I didn't mind applying some coconut oil on his back. He put on an old T-shirt in case all of the oil did not soak in. After about thirty minutes, he said it felt much better and went to take a nap.

I have read that people can soak their feet in a solution made with cornmeal and very warm water to stop fungus of the toenails, etc. This solution was said to work because corn has anti-fungal properties to protect itself from disease. I think the baking soda in warm water might be effective for this also, but we have not had occasion to try it.

Fever Blisters (Cold Sores)

The National Institute of Health says that herpes simplex virus type 1 affects about 20% of children age five, 60% of people in their thirties, and over 85% of old people.

Last year I had a chance to try the concept of letting alcohol soak into the skin to stop a fever blister. The unmistakable tingling sensation and bump was about a quarter-inch below my mouth. Since I was really serious about wanting to stop it, I used 70% rubbing alcohol on a swab and held it on the bump, until I noticed that it felt like a cold spot coming to the inside of my mouth. That actually did shut it down immediately. Within hours it was totally gone!

I don't advise putting 70% isopropyl alcohol on your skin, even though it is commonly used in hand cleaners and other personal products. I certainly wouldn't put it on my lips or in my mouth, since that is not recommended by the Texas Poison Control Center. But I wouldn't hesitate to try diluted or even full-strength vodka on a cotton swab to kill such a virus—now that I know alcohol will put a stop to it. Dabbing it on does not work. You have to keep the spot wet long enough to let it soak in.

Recently, I read that the same virus that causes cold sores on the mouth can contribute to Alzheimer's or dementia; and it is best to treat fever blisters as quickly as possible, to make the virus return to the dormant stage.

Poison Ivy

This is the opposite of a transdermal treatment. The culprit is attacking you transdermally, while the answer is simply to remove it.

I learned to identify poison ivy at a young age. I played Tarzan and Jane with neighborhood kids on a lot that was overgrown with trees and vines. Fortunately, I didn't get a rash; but my sister got a terrible case of poison ivy. Calamine lotion provided little relief for the misery that she experienced.

After I was married, I decided to remove some poison ivy which was growing under a small shrub, because it was a constant threat to anyone doing yard work. I wore gloves, of course, and even wrapped vinyl around it while pulling it out; but that wasn't adequate. If I ever had immunity, I didn't any more. There was no effective remedy that I could find, and it had to run its course. The best advice was to use Calamine lotion and not to scratch. The first piece of advice really doesn't help much. The second is hard to follow, especially when you are asleep.

If you have never had poison ivy, just believe me when I say it is the most intense itch I have ever experienced. It is not contagious, but it can be spread if the offending oil (urushiol) is on your hands or garden tools. I avoid burning any plant materials mixed with poison ivy, because it is said that breathing the smoke can be especially harmful.

During the 1980s, we lived across the street from the Big Thicket in East Texas with our two active boys. We eradicated poison ivy from our property; but, if the boys chased a ball or petted the family dog, it was back to haunt us. A dermatologist prescribed an ointment that reduced inflammation and anesthetized the itch. It was rather expensive but provided precious relief. We would cut the tube to get out the last tiny bit.

That product was taken off the market some years later because of safety issues. I think there was a problem with people using it on broken skin. We were advised to scrub with bath soap immediately after exposure. That helped some, if you knew you had been exposed. But common knowledge still said there was no cure.

New products came out later. One was a wash that was supposed to be used before contact. Good luck. Another was a cream that could be obtained over the counter. It contained tiny, glassy beads that would help remove the urushiol when massaged over the skin. Forty-five dollars was the biggest price I had ever paid for an over-the-counter product; but I could get it without a visit to the dermatologist, and it worked.

After urushiol contacts your skin, it may take a day or two for the reaction to manifest itself. By that time, it's too late to stop it with commercial soap. But wait! There is an old-time remedy that really works.

Here is the protocol: Use a terry-type wash cloth to scrub the area with Grandma's Lye Soap, and then rinse well. It's a scrumptious way to soothe the itch and wash yourself free of the wicked oil that causes so much misery. This works even after the rash has appeared—if you don't let it go too long. It's okay to wash with lye soap several times, if necessary, until you know you have removed all traces of the offending oil. The itching will stop as soon as you get your skin really clean.

Don't roll your eyes at me! Many people are afraid of lye soap. They tell stories of how it burns or that homemade soap looks brown and dirty, etc. They are not describing properly-made lye soap. They also tell about how grandma washed out their mouth with soap after a naughty word. Please don't blame that on lye soap.

The first fact to make clear is that all bar soap is made with an alkali and some kind of fat which, when cooked together, saponify or turn to soap. Real lye soap has had nothing removed and does not contain any additives. It is, in fact, very gentle to the skin. I have read that glycerin is removed from commercial soaps because it can be sold separately for more money. You might not even want to know how many additives are used in commercial soaps.

The good news is that Grandma's Lye Soap is made in Oklahoma and contains nothing but lye, lard, and water. The cost is about $5.00 for a nice-sized bar. No, I don't own any stock in the business that makes it. Don't buy the copycat product which is made in China and contains additives.

You can also find real homemade soap at farmer's markets, craft or gift shops, and local farm stores. Some might even be made with olive oil or Shea butter. But each one is also made from some sort of lye or ashes. I haven't tried the other variations. I heard recently that Grandma's Lye Soap now offers a bar that is especially for poison ivy, but I have not tried it either.

A friend told me that the lye soap didn't work for him. After further discussion, it turned out that he had used it on a landscape job where a sink was not available. He had used his water jug to wet his hands and lather with the soap, then poured a little more water to rinse. The missing link was that the skin must be scrubbed with the lye soap to remove the urushiol before rinsing thoroughly. A further caution is that if the water jug and tool handles have been contaminated with urushiol, they must be scrubbed also, before using them again.

Since urushiol is invisible, it is impossible to tell if you got it all off after exposure; but it is not too late when you realize a reaction is starting. Repeat the scrubbing with lye soap until all itching stops. Don't just give up and let it break out.

It is heartbreaking to think about all the suffering that has been caused by these plants, when such a simple and inexpensive solution exists.

At our present home, there is more poison ivy in the woods than I have ever seen in one spot. It constantly comes back to areas we have cleared. But I don't have to be afraid of it any more. I just dig it up with a small shovel, or whatever tool is at hand, and toss it into the edge of the woods, or any place where I am not currently working. I know not to touch the blade of the shovel until it has been used sufficiently in soil to wear off any remaining oil.

If a rash is oozing because you didn't get to the lye soap in time, our cousin reports that you can wrap it in gauze soaked in an Epsom salts solution. That would be a transdermal treatment.

In closing this chapter, I must say that it would behoove you to be aware of what is coming through your skin. Is behoove still a word? Well, I did tell you I am a grandma.

Chapter 5
Other Insights

Sinusitis

Now that you know how to defend yourself against colds and allergies, I need to talk a little more about sinusitis. Although our chances of having sinusitis are greatly reduced while we are avoiding colds and allergies, it is still possible for infections to start in the sinuses.

Back in the days before I discovered Dr. Judd's advice, I had no trouble recognizing a sinus infection. I spent many days coughing, blowing my nose, and taking antihistamines. This would be followed by pressure around my eyes and cheeks, fever, and thick green or yellow mucus. There was no mistake. Now I have to be alert for more subtle symptoms.

Since I am able to avoid any congestion and medication, the first sign of sinusitis might be a slight headache around my eyes or teeth, or a warm feeling on my cheeks. If sniffing a drop of diluted vodka doesn't take care of it, I go ahead and do the salt water thing. If any thick mucus comes out, I know I didn't waste my time. Then I follow up with extra vitamin C to fight it off. So the thing to remember is that you have to be more perceptive to detect the first clues, but you can easily stop a sinus infection before the symptoms get even more obvious.

I recently discovered a 1999 press release from Mayo Clinic, which adds some further insight to our defense strategy. The researchers stated that an immune system response to *fungus*—rather than bacteria—is responsible for about 96% of chronic sinusitis. They further advised that the usual treatment with antibiotics and steroids could actually destroy the body's natural defenses and make fungal proliferation more likely.

Can you see another Grandma's remedy coming on here? In some of the recipes for sniffing salt water that I have seen on the Internet, they said to add a pinch of baking soda along with the 1/2 teaspoon of salt for each cup of water, to make it more comfortable.

Baking soda is exactly the remedy I discovered for fungal infections on the skin. If I ever get another sinus infection, I will certainly add a pinch of baking soda to the heated water for sniffing. It might even be as important as the salt. We will have to fine-tune our own recipes.

The Mayo Clinic, of course, recommended that you see an ear, nose, and throat specialist who is familiar with their recommendations for treating fungal sinusitis, if home remedies are not successful. I second that.

Toxic Fumes

In June of 2012 I was working in an office where I do bookkeeping. Suddenly the room was filled with solvent fumes from a remodeling job in the space above. Since we have no operable windows, I went upstairs to ask if they could provide better exhaust ventilation—to no avail. So we called the building manager to put in our request, propped our hallway door open, and went back to work.

A short time later, I could feel a little dry sensation in the upper reaches of my nostrils and a slight feeling of pressure in my head, the unmistakable sign that I had an allergy headache coming on. Since our office is one of the first in the USA to be stocked with cotton swabs and a bottle of mouthwash, I didn't have to go out to my car to manage a nip-it trick. Even though the fumes were still strong in the air, I felt a slight drainage a few minutes later, letting me know that the headache had been averted. Although I was free to leave, I went back to work.

The contractor appeared later, apologized profusely, and corrected the problems upstairs. I tried to keep working, but I began to realize that I was skipping entries and marking items as posted in the wrong column. I finally came to my senses enough to know that I needed to go to lunch an hour early to get some fresh air.

Here are some lessons from my experience:

- I should not tolerate toxic fumes when wearing my book-keeper hat, any more than when wearing my homebuilder hat.
- Mouthwash or 14% alcohol is effective at stopping allergic headaches, even against toxic fumes that are still in the air. This surprised even me!
- Since toxic fumes can be absorbed by our lungs, our eyes, and even our biggest organ, our skin, the only real remedy is to escape.

Vitamin E

I will not be discussing vitamin A, the B vitamins, etc., although they are important to our health. I am focusing on vitamins C and D. But vitamin E does need to be mentioned, because it has received some undeserved negative publicity. Appendix E is an editorial that can set the record straight.

Fluoride

For many years, I have been concerned about fluoridation of public water supplies. I have never found any convincing evidence that the benefits outweigh the dangers. Since there is no daily requirement for fluoride as a nutrient, I can't imagine why we should be drinking it. From all indications I can find, it is more likely to cause brittle bones than to prevent tooth decay. I don't think it is a coincidence that I have had no cracked teeth since I started avoiding fluoride as much as possible.

I recently saw a video on YouTube, demonstrating that the ten largest US cities with fluoridation have a much higher cancer rate than the ten largest cities without it. Also, I have heard from numerous sources that fluoride can decrease children's IQ.

Having been involved in fluoride research, Dr. Judd was adamant that it should not be added to drinking water. He even recommended avoiding any toothpaste and using soap instead. He said bar soap would clean the teeth well and rinse away more easily than toothpaste.

Appendix F is an editorial worth sharing.

Supplements in General

The three news releases that make up Appendix G are included to emphasize the safety and necessity of vitamin supplements. The third one even contains suggestions for how you might participate in furthering the cause of nutritional medicine. I am encouraged by the progress that is being made.

Bacteria Are Us

This is an extremely vast and important topic; but I just need to mention it briefly here, in case you are not familiar with it.

In 2003 I was introduced to the *Soil Food Web* at a native plant conference. For most of my life, gardening organically just meant using compost and mulch, and avoiding poisons and chemicals. But here on a big screen was the whole story of what is going on beneath our feet—how a teaspoon of healthy soil is full of millions of microbes, including bacteria, fungi, and other critters that have a synergistic relationship with the plants and provide nutrients in exchange for the sugars that plants make through photosynthesis. Everything eats something else, not all nematodes are bad, microbes also live inside the plants, and so forth.

We have always been told that plants don't know the difference between natural or synthetic fertilizers, as if that somehow justifies the lifeless soils across our country. For more information about real soil, see the *Soil Biology Primer,* available through the online store of the Soil and Water Conservation Service.

Well, guess what, folks? The same applies to us! Only about 10% of the cells in our body are of human origin. The rest are bacteria, fungi, and who knows what else. While they represent far less than 90% of our weight, the roles they play in our existence are still being discovered and may never be fully understood. I know this might be shocking, if you have not heard it before—but just ask any microbiologist.

The next question is, what have we been doing to the fungus among us, not to mention the bacteria? Well, let's see. Antibiotics kill bacteria, not all bacteria are bad, and the details of our synergistic existence are still being discovered.

For example, H. pylori was linked with stomach ulcers; so it has been widely eradicated with antibiotics. Now we are learning that it also has beneficial uses, like assisting hormones in the stomach that tell us when we are full. Could that be a little clue to some of our obesity problems? It also is believed to have a role in preventing esophageal cancer, asthma, and other conditions.

H. pylori is just one of many hundreds of species of bacteria that live in our gastrointestinal tract, most of which have not yet been identified, not to mention the numerous microbes that occupy other parts of our bodies.

In studying the soil food web, I learned that trees and perennials like fungi-dominated soils, while vegetables, annuals, and grasses prefer more bacteria. What do antibiotics do for the balance of fungi and bacteria in our bodies? I just know that antibiotics can have a negative effect on our digestion and are not appropriate for most chronic sinus infections, as mentioned above.

According to several health newsletters which I have received recently, our metabolic pathways are a series of chemical reactions our bodies perform to stay alive. Since the role that microbes play in our metabolic pathways is still unfolding, we really don't know how many species of microbes may be critical to our existence. We can expect to hear a lot more about new discoveries regarding invisible friends and foes.

We have become almost obsessed with sterilizing our floors, hands, and even babies. Now we are learning that some of the healthiest children have been inoculated through mother's milk, gradual introduction to grass and soil, etc. It is time to realize that not all bacteria are bad, and some are even beneficial. Antibacterial products are not the answer for everything.

I couldn't be happier that I don't get secondary respiratory infections any more, since that has always been the main reason I had to use antibiotics. If I do begin to get a sore throat or other signs of a cold, I can stop it with a drop of diluted alcohol, rather than more drastic measures. It occurs to me that Dr. Judd has made a significant contribution toward enabling us to reduce our use of antibiotics.

Sunshine

So what else is new? What about decades of misinformation about the dangers of sunshine. While sunburn is, of course, to be avoided, we have been misled into widespread deficiencies of vitamin D.

I figured out that Santa Clause thing when I was six, but now I find that I have been misinformed all my life about C and D—two of the vitamins most critical to our health.

Chapter 6
Vitamin C—More Than Meets the Eye

On February 1, 2012, before 8:00 p.m., a large meteorite was seen over Odessa and Abilene, Texas. It exploded over Dallas and fell somewhere within about a hundred miles east of Dallas. It was a spectacular fireball, estimated to weigh over 1,000 pounds before breaking up. Marble-sized pieces would have fallen first, with the largest pieces cratering into the ground further east. Many witnesses said it was the most impressive thing they had ever seen.

But guess what? Most people in the area didn't even know it happened. They might have been at home with drapes drawn, watching television. Maybe a farmer has already filled in what he thought was an armadillo hole. Since rocks from the sky belong to the land owner (unlike pieces of space debris that belong to the government), the farmer might have buried a treasure, without seeing it, or sharing it with scientists who are searching for a way to prevent future asteroid impacts. But unless a big space rock nicks your roof and spares your life, while making you wealthy, you really don't need to know the details about a fireball.

Ever since the discovery of vitamin C in the 1930s, however, its importance to mankind is a story that somehow continues to go right over our heads! We all know that we need vitamin C to prevent scurvy. But there is much more to it than that. Despite all the new supplements coming onto the market, vitamin C could well be the most important supplement we can take.

Most mammals manufacture their own vitamin C. The only known exceptions are apes, guinea pigs, bats, and humans. Generally, the heavier the animal, the more vitamin C it produces. Based on other mammals, a 150-pound man should produce about 4000 mg per day. It has been demonstrated that healthy people may not need that much on a daily basis, but those with illness would need much more.

I had known for a long time that the trait of not producing vitamin C was what guinea pigs had in common with humans. That was why they were used in some scientific experiments rather than rats. When I decided to research it further, it got more interesting. It turns out that we have a genetic defect that makes us incapable of making our own vitamin C like all other mammals on earth, with the exception of the few species mentioned above. In 1959 a biochemist isolated it to a mutation in a specific gene.

Most species make vitamin C in their liver out of glucose, by using four enzymes. We make the first three enzymes that are required; but although we come that close, the fourth one, gulonolactone oxidase enzyme, is absent because of a defect in a certain gene. Apparently, it is not known how or when this mutation could have occurred.

The few animals that cannot produce vitamin C all have a plant diet that can provide ascorbate; but man's diet might not, especially in the coldest climates. This brings up the question of how we have survived so well without adequate vitamin C. Maybe some of us didn't.

Early man, who foraged for food, is thought to have consumed over 600 mg of vitamin C per day. Today we are said to consume only about 110 mg. from the average diet. Our modern processed foods may have some vitamins added; but unless we are gardeners, most fruits and vegetables get to us in less than optimum condition. Our love of cooking causes vitamin C to be destroyed as well, so it is likely that some people may not be getting even that much.

One thought-provoking observation is that animals that produce their own vitamin C tend to live eight or more times their age at maturity, while we live only about four times our age at maturity. This hints that our lack of adequate vitamin C might well have more impact than we thought, in regard to aging and disease.

I wonder if our tendency to develop diabetes might have been alleviated somewhat if we were capable of transforming some of our blood sugar into vitamin C, like other species. I have a lot of questions, but my solution is to try to take enough vitamin C to protect my health.

Dr. Linus Pauling discovered that ascorbate is used up in the making of collagen, which is what maintains the structural integrity of connective tissue, skin, and blood vessels. Our arterial walls are more delicate and more subject to damage than those of other mammals. Regeneration is impossible without adequate collagen. Our arteries begin to deteriorate in areas of the most stress, then plaque forms on weak spots to prevent leaks. Dr. Pauling found that there is a 3.5 times greater risk of heart attack among men who are ascorbate deficient, than those who are not.

Due to its shorter life span, a guinea pig that is denied vitamin C will have heart disease within weeks. Animals that do manufacture their own vitamin C can apparently make quite large amounts when their body is subject to disease or other stress. Among those animals, there appears to be no incidence of heart disease.

I read many years ago that the government's recommended daily allowance (RDA) of vitamin C was only adequate to prevent scurvy, and that blaming cholesterol for heart disease was like blaming a fireman who came to a fire. Without enough collagen available, the body sends cholesterol to repair the damage; so it gets blamed for causing the problem. Only with extra vitamin C can the body provide enough collagen for the damage to be repaired properly. There is abundant evidence that hardening of the arteries or coronary heart disease is nothing more than chronic arterial scurvy!

Although some have claimed that large amounts of vitamin C are ill advised, other researchers recommend taking about 4,000 mg on a daily basis and increasing to as much as 15,000 mg or more, when needed to fight illness. Vitamin C has also been accused of causing kidney stones and vitamin B12 deficiency, but this has been proven false. Another issue was whether ascorbic acid could be strong enough to damage tooth enamel, but that can be avoided by rinsing the teeth with plain water.

If more vitamin C is taken orally than can be absorbed, it will result in diarrhea. The method of adjusting large doses to bowel tolerance involves consuming plenty of pure water and decreasing, but not stopping the vitamin C, when it appears that level is about to be reached.

Dr. Pauling felt that a daily dose of vitamin C, just under the amount to cause looseness of the bowel, would be best for fighting many diseases, including colon cancer. He took about 18,000 mg every day and lived to be over 90. He criticized the U.S. Government's RDA, saying it was based on the known amount to prevent acute scurvy, but not the dosage needed for optimal health.

Even today the RDA for vitamin C in the United States is 90 mg for an adult male and 75 mg for an adult female! The tolerable upper intake level for either is said to be 2,000 mg per day. I suppose that could be true if you are more concerned about the possibility of diarrhea than the numerous rampant diseases and conditions that could be prevented or even reversed with vitamin C.

There appears to be no significant difference in the bioavailability of natural versus synthetic ascorbic acid. Slow-release preparations have not been found to have any advantage either—although it is best to spread doses through the day. Vitamin C buffered with baking soda (sodium ascorbate) is more palatable than plain ascorbic acid.

I was concerned that taking megadoses of sodium ascorbate might result in consuming too much sodium; but then I learned that the sodium which is known for raising blood pressure is sodium chloride and that sodium ascorbate should not adversely affect hypertension. I have seen no problem with it, but that is something which should be determined individually.

Some physicians are administering intravenous as well as intramuscular ascorbate with impressive results, although hospitals in the United States do not allow these procedures. If you would like to have these treatments available to you when needed, it is recommended that you locate a doctor or clinic in advance.

Vitamin C is a natural anti-inflammatory, with more potential than we realize. It has been used successfully in megadoses to stop multiple chemical sensitivity (MCS) and many other reactions to toxins.

Dr. Tom Levy has written that Vitamin C is "the best broad-spectrum antibiotic, antihistamine, antitoxic and antiviral substance there is." He also said it has been proven capable of quickly curing acute polio and acute hepatitis. Other viral diseases it can cure and prevent include AIDS, chickenpox, influenza, measles, mumps, and rabies. Non-viral infectious diseases which can be cured include diphtheria, leprosy, malaria, strep, tetanus, tuberculosis, and typhoid fever. There are also long lists of pathogenic microorganisms and even toxins, such as mushroom poisoning, which can be successfully treated. For a lot more information than I can mention, I recommend his most recent book *Primal Panacea*, by Thomas E. Levy, M.D., J.D. Since he is a cardiologist, you might also be interested in his conclusion that "Vitamin C deficiency in the coronary arteries is the *solitary root cause* of all coronary heart disease."

A recent report claimed that Japanese workers, who underwent a high-dose vitamin C treatment before exposure to severe radiation at Fukushima, were protected against DNA damage and cancer. They were given 25,000 mg. of intravenous vitamin C and oral antioxidants, like alpha-lipoic acid and vitamin E. Similar follow-up treatments were provided to workers who did not receive advance protection, and after two months they were found to have their free DNA levels and cancer scores returned to normal.

If you can't believe you read the previous few paragraphs correctly, please read them again. I think it is time for us to demand the right to use vitamin C in whatever doses and whatever forms of treatment are needed and to persuade our physicians to become familiar with the impressive science behind vitamin C.

Please see Appendix C.5 for an important news release by Dr. Levy about what we need to know to stand up for our rights as patients and to bring our medical care into the 21st Century.

Liposomal Vitamin C is another type which is now available. This is an oral form of vitamin C encased in microscopic, fluid-filled bubbles made of phospholipids similar to cell membranes. Liposomes can deliver substances to the blood so efficiently that absorption might approach 90%, rather than the typical 10% or so. This form is, of course, more expensive than tablets; but you would have to consider the efficiency and convenience as compared to the cost per dose.

A friend of mine had purchased a supply of liposomal C in small packets and had occasion to use some of them when her son got a nasty cut on his arm. As soon as they noticed a red streak starting up his arm, she called his doctor and got an appointment for 11:00 a.m. She started giving him a dose every hour, and by the time they saw the doctor, the streak was actually receding. They accepted the prescription for antibiotics, but did not have to fill it. I think liposomal C would be a great product to have in a first aid kit. It is also good for treatment of any of the above-listed diseases, if you cannot arrange for vitamin C injections or IV's when needed.

Getting back to the subject of taking 4000 mg of vitamin C on a daily basis, we found that it was not easy to do. Eight 500 mg tablets are entirely too many for us, since we also take other supplements; so I keep some larger tablets on hand for my husband. I prefer more of the powder forms. Plain ascorbic acid powder is inexpensive and easy to incorporate into drinks; but it is rather sour, since I prefer not to add sugar or other sweeteners.

I find the sodium ascorbate easy to use, by keeping it in a sugar dispenser that can drop a half teaspoon at a time into a small amount of water. I swirl it in the bottom of the glass until dissolved, then fill the glass with cold filtered water. Since the ascorbate is buffered and the water contains no fluoride or chlorine, the taste is not too bad. It is somewhere between water with lemon and plain water. I sip it for an hour or two while working at my desk or watching television, so I can possibly benefit by consuming it over a longer period of time. The dispenser is also handy for adding a measured amount to a bottle of water to take outdoors or in the car. The taste is really not even noticeable in juice or smoothies.

The liposomal packets of vitamin C are good to keep on hand for emergencies, since I have not found a source for injection or I.V.

in our area. I found some liposomal vitamin C on amazon.com, although it was not yet available locally.

One of the criticisms of liposomal products was that they didn't taste good. We have learned to put about a quarter to a half-inch of water in a small condiment cup and squeeze the packet contents into it. Then it can be swallowed quite easily, without noticing much taste at all, since the water prevents it from clinging to the tongue or throat. This is a way to get a lot more vitamin C into the blood than taking tablets, and it is so well-absorbed that it does not cause flushing of the bowel. One thousand milligrams from one packet is apparently capable of putting about 900 mg into the blood stream, while you would have to take about nine 1000 mg tablets to have the same benefit.

I just wish I had discovered the significance of my real shortage of vitamin C years ago, so that I would be much further down the road in preventing cataracts, heart disease, and all of the other diseases and conditions mentioned above. It is sad that most of us are struggling along with deficiencies—unaware that such an easy and inexpensive preventative exists.

Unfortunately, many doctors have had very little training in nutrition; yet I have known people who would not take a vitamin or eat an egg, unless their doctor said they could. I have had some success in sharing information about vitamins or probiotics with my physicians in the past, but sometimes I just have to find a more tolerant doctor.

Although there are many thousands of deaths per year in the United States because of prescription drugs—and almost none which can be blamed on vitamins—our government seems determined to regulate how much vitamin C and other critically important supplements we can take. I wish they were as determined to control (or at least label) genetically modified foods.

I don't want to advise you to do anything that has been deemed illegal. You will need to decide how much vitamin C is best for you, after doing your own research. I think you will agree that there is much more to it than meets the eye.

Although the original concept came from Jeremiah 5:21 of the King James Version, I can still hear the old saying, "There are none as blind as those who will not see."

Chapter 7
Vitamin D3—A New Look

Most of what is known about vitamin D was just learned in the past ten or fifteen years. Our needs are actually much greater than previously believed. Due to false assumptions about sun exposure and low nutritional recommendations, it is said that 85% of the American public and about 95% of senior citizens are deficient.

Now we are told that sunshine actually helps prevent cancer. It is only over-exposure and sunburn that cause problems. I had my share of both as a teenager.

After having basal cell carcinoma on my nose in the 1970s, I had been advised to always wear long sleeves, a big hat, and sun block. As soon as I read about the new discoveries regarding vitamin D, I knew this was important information for me. Although by this time I was eating free-range eggs and my own organic vegetables, I knew I had to be deficient.

I started taking 5,000 IU of D3 per day and noticed that my skin improved, my eyes didn't feel dry anymore, and my wrist pain vanished. I don't know how low my blood level had been; but when I later got my first test, my serum blood level was at 35. I switched to taking 10,000 IU per day and in six months my level had improved to 51. After averaging 7500 IU for the next six months, my blood level was 61. Now I try to maintain my level between 50 and 70 for optimal health.

The brand of D3 that we use comes in 5,000 and 10,000 IU. When I fill our little boxes marked for the days of the week, I put one strength in every other compartment and then fill in with the other size. This is more economical than taking more pearls of a lesser potency to equal 7,500 IU per day. If we should find that we can decrease our dosage even more, we will further reduce the frequency of taking 10,000 IU.

Let me back up and explain some of the above figures. The only way we can know for sure if we are getting enough vitamin D is to get a blood test. The ideal blood level is now said by the Vitamin D Council to be 50 to 70 Nano grams per milliliter, rather than the old baseline of 25 for rickets prevention. Research indicates that blood levels between 70 and 100 can be beneficial for those fighting disease, but levels above 100 could be toxic.

Unlike the water soluble vitamins which are measured in grams (g), milligrams (mg), or even micrograms (mcg), the oily vitamins are measured in international units (IU). While water soluble vitamins that are not absorbed pass easily through the body, the fat soluble ones could possibly be accumulated to excess—hence the need for occasional testing.

Vitamin D can prevent many diseases. It is now said to be more of a hormone, rather than a vitamin. It regulates 10% of our DNA and can cut our risk of cancer by as much as 50%. I think you will agree that just taking enough D3 to prevent rickets is far from adequate.

It has been discovered that taking 35 to 40 IU per pound of body weight per day is effective against seventeen types of cancer, as well as heart disease, hypertension, autoimmune diseases, diabetes, depression, osteoporosis, chronic pain, muscle weakness, birth defects, periodontal disease, and many other diseases and conditions. This would be a dose of 6,000 IU per day for a 150-pound adult, just as an example.

All children need a proper level to form good teeth and bones, as well as to boost immunity. A fifty-pound child can take 2,000 IU per day and prevent a lot more than rickets.

Senior citizens are said to be the most deficient. Improved levels have been found to relieve pain, as well as prevent falls, broken bones, and much more.

Infants are deficient also. It had been assumed that babies didn't need much, because there is practically no vitamin D in human breast milk; but it turned out that this has only been true because most lactating women are deficient.

There are some terrible stories in this country about breastfed babies being removed from their natural parents because of broken bones or other perceived abuse. Actually, these babies were so deficient in vitamin D that they had rickets or similar conditions with bones soft enough to be damaged just through normal daily care. Then when they were placed in foster care and given commercial formulas containing a minimal amount of vitamin D, their condition might improve enough to appear that they were no longer being abused. Without a prior test for vitamin D, it could be impossible to prove that there was no intentional abuse. It seems to me that any baby suspected of being abused, but without bruises, should immediately be tested for vitamin D before other formulas are given.

It is shocking that an infant blessed enough to be fed naturally by its mother could be so severely harmed by a deficiency in her diet. Maybe a Serum25(OH)D test could be done soon after birth, if they are drawing blood at that time anyway; or pregnant women should be advised about the need for adequate vitamin D3. More education is definitely needed.

The broader picture is that our whole society is deficient in vitamin D, but when researchers presented the information to the authorities they refused to increase their recommendations to reasonable amounts. They did increase the amount somewhat for babies, but not for adults.

Some researchers say that almost any adult should be able to take 10,000 IU of D3 per day for two weeks. If you see any improvement in your health and comfort, you should take time to get a Serum25(OH)D test, to see how much you can take to optimize your health. If I had it to do over, I would want to know how deficient I was before supplementing, just to satisfy my curiosity.

Sunlight is a natural source, but for most of the year it is difficult to get enough. The further from the equator you live, the greater chance you have of being deficient. Also, the darker your skin, the more difficult it is to absorb enough.

The early morning and later afternoon hours, which used to be recommended for avoiding sunburn, are now known to provide only the UVA rays that can cause cancer. The same is true of cloudy or overcast days. UVB light is the wave length needed for vitamin D production. I remember that by telling myself that the B stands for "best."

Getting sunlight on large areas of your skin for 15 minutes without sun block on a clear day can equal 10,000 units. That is a little clue if you are concerned that taking 10,000 IU might be too risky. I have read that five to 35 minutes per day, three times per week between 10 a.m. and 3 p.m. might provide enough to maintain good health. That sounds easy enough. However, most Americans are at work or school during those hours of the day and are not dressed for sun bathing.

After UVB rays on the skin cause a cholesterol derivative to be converted to vitamin D3, it takes up to 24 hours or more to be absorbed. Unfortunately, if you bathe with soap in the meantime, it may be washed away first. How many of us want to wait that long to take a good bath after being out in the sun?

One suggestion is to avoid lathering up large areas of skin which have just been exposed to sunlight. I don't know about you, but I will have to rely on vitamin D3. I don't want to discourage anyone from getting their vitamin D free from the sun, however, because some researchers think there could be additional benefits not yet discovered.

Tanning equipment with the right type of rays can actually be beneficial, while other units should be avoided. Just remember that you only want UVB rays. A similar warning is that sunlight through glass should be avoided, because only the beneficial UVB rays are filtered out.

Even lifeguards or others who get plenty of vitamin D from sunshine in the summer may need to take supplements during the winter.

Vitamin D2 should be avoided. Although it might still be used for prescriptions and in many food products, it is actually poorly absorbed. By law it is added to milk, but not to milk products.

Vegetables can be a source of natural vitamin D, but they don't contain very much. Milk and cheese have very little. Oily fish may contain the most. Supplementation of vitamin D3, rather than cod-liver oil, can help prevent colds and flu and might even be a good alternative to flu shots.

One of my best friends was seeing a doctor for osteopenia and pain, until they finally did a blood test and found that her vitamin D level was only 16. I was really surprised because she was very tanned and athletic, but it just shows that you can't really tell without proper testing. Her doctor prescribed huge amounts of D2, because that was all that was available for prescriptions at the time.

Vitamin D3 has now become available in units of 50,000 IU, which can be prescribed to be taken once a week. As an alternative, you might decide to take 10,000 IU every day until a test shows a proper level, since it is inexpensive and does not require a prescription. Then you can determine what daily amount is needed to maintain that level with less frequent testing.

For more information, see Appendix D.1 through D.5. To follow the latest vitamin D research, see http://www.vitamindcouncil.org.

Chapter 8
Parting Thoughts

Health Records

If you leave all of your medical records in the care of your physician, you might lose much of the history when you move or the doctor closes his practice, etc. Why not put yourself in charge?

Say you have changed jobs or moved to a new area. After all insurance claims have been settled, those records can be discarded. But first, you might want to go through and make a little log of dates and whatever matters were addressed. I always save test results and any X-rays. I have learned to ask for these, because I found that if they were requested later they might no longer be available. I also list any medications and the period of time they were taken. It is good to keep all documentation of vaccinations—so they won't have to be taken again for lack of proof.

I remember several times over the years having respiratory complications, just when the weather had warmed up and people weren't as likely to be sick. It wasn't until I looked over my log and noticed how many times I had serious secondary infections in March, that I realized these were probably triggered by a pollen that comes out at that time of year.

Keep a few notes between appointments with your doctor if you notice any minor changes in your condition or if you make any changes in your routine or diet that may be relevant, etc. You can take your file to each appointment to assist in updating the doctor on your progress, and it can serve as a good reference if you change doctors or need emergency care. Some people find it helpful to make a list of questions before visits, and then jot down all the doctor's instructions.

If you should decide to start maximizing your use of vitamins C, D, or any other supplement, it might be worthwhile to make a note of any symptoms you are experiencing when you start. Your notes could be helpful in comparing your results later. I know that for us, we tend to forget little problems after they disappear and don't even notice they are gone.

About ten years ago, my husband had been told by an excellent orthopedic physician that he would need a knee replacement soon. I put the little educational brochure the assistant had given us into our medical file and hoped Medicare and supplemental insurance would take care of it when the time came. Subsequently, I modified my diet to stop symptoms of inflammation; and, by default, his diet was changed somewhat also. Then we went into an extensive do-it-yourself project, building our eco-farm. It wasn't until I was doing research for this chapter, that I came across the little brochure in the file. I went running to find him and ask about the status of his knee. He was as astonished as I was, because he had totally forgotten about it. I guess we tend to take good things for granted!

Research

If you have an ongoing medical condition, it would be worthwhile to become your own expert. No matter how diligent your doctor is at keeping up with medical advances, no one can know everything. If you are self-informed, your doctor won't have to spend extra time educating you about the basics, and you can ask more meaningful questions.

You might want to make a little file for each condition or disease that runs in your family. If a parent died of a stroke, you might want to make a folder to save anything that appears in publications about the latest discoveries and treatments. Save a list inside the front of the file that shows tests for various symptoms of stroke—not that you will have time to look it up if you are stricken, but because you will see it occasionally when filing. Since medical attention should be sought as quickly as possible, determine which hospital is best equipped and closest to your home. Maybe a different one is closer to your place of work. Then if that dreaded time ever comes, 911 can be dialed; and you will know which hospital you prefer if there is a choice. Even better, maybe you can learn to avoid the pitfalls that lead to a particular condition.

If anyone if your family ever breaks a bone, you will want to know in advance which orthopedic specialist to request. It can make a difference.

Some people don't subscribe to newspapers anymore and rely on numerous electronic devices. While technology is more convenient, it is easier to overlook important local issues and new advances in health and wellness. Too many television news programs are about a murder thousands of miles away or the latest personal problems of a celebrity, rather than information that is important to our lives. But we can still learn about new discoveries from numerous sources.

The Internet is our most valuable resource for research—from top scientific studies to blogs by people looking for answers. Just be careful out there. The most impressive research projects don't always start with honest criteria, and some of the blogs contain remedies that can be outright dangerous. So consider the source, and check for numerous other opinions.

Wikipedia can be a source for general information. It can provide an overview of many subjects, compared to the jungle of websites. But keep in mind that it is written by contributors all over the world, and that some opinions express vested interests.

The fact that a website is considered a medical source does not mean that everything they say is correct. For example, I noticed a site just recently with a video using the slang word for mucus. They said it is really a good thing, and if you are congested for a few days it is nothing to worry about! I don't want to mention any names, but their initials are WebMD. I promise that's my last little jest.

If you have had a chance to try the tips I have described, you know that staying free of congestion is essential to staying well.

Recipe Ideas

Since most conventional mouthwashes contain artificial colors and sweeteners, along with other questionable ingredients, I tried to come up with a recipe to include in the appendices to make diluted vodka more pleasant. I thought it would be good to have a hint of beneficial essential oils for flavor, a touch of xylitol or stevia for the sweetener (if needed), and maybe a trace of some natural coloring, so it would not look like plain water. Organic vodka could be used for the 14% alcohol. Organic glycerin is available also, but I don't know what amount would be beneficial or whether it would be just as effective without it.

I experimented with several ideas, but I was not happy with my results. Some had great scent and flavor, but just didn't live up to my expectations. It is very easy to dilute vodka as described in Appendix B; but adding optional ingredients, such as those suggested above, requires more expertise.

For example, in one of my experiments, I thought it would be a great idea to add a little vitamin C. So I put one-fourth teaspoon of sodium ascorbate into a three-ounce bottle of diluted vodka while waiting for my order of essential oils to come in. The two-week wait was beneficial, because I learned something important. The liquid gradually changed color from clear to a rich amber. Since no other ingredients had been added yet, I realized that the vitamin C had oxidized, making it useless. In fact, it would have had a negative effect because oxidized vitamin C becomes something the body has to eliminate, along with any toxins. So the lesson to keep in mind is that vitamin C should not be diluted for very long before it is used. I don't know how they stabilize the liquid forms of vitamin C to preserve effectiveness.

Comments about Alcohol

It seems to be common knowledge that alcohol is drying to the mouth and throat. The only problem is—I don't know where people got that knowledge. While a tiny bit of alcohol can halt histamine reactions and can even stop an allergic headache while the irritant is still present, I must agree with Dr. Judd's opinion that diluted alcohol is a good wetting agent and can help normalize the nasal passages. I speak from experience, because I have been using it for the past eight years to stop all colds, respiratory allergies, and headaches, and even to soothe a dry nose in the winter. That common knowledge—that alcohol is drying—is simply incorrect in regard to using diluted alcohol as an occasional remedy in the nose and throat; and it needs to go the way of our false beliefs about vitamin D and sunshine.

I do have some concern about recommending the use of vodka. During my impressionable years, I got the impression that alcohol wasn't for me. This was reinforced when I was about eighteen. An acquaintance in a nearby town asked me to come over early and help her get ready for a party. While we were preparing snacks, she offered me some citrus punch which had been mixed by someone before I arrived. It was delicious. I even had a second serving. Then I started feeling ill, before more guests arrived, and decided I needed to go home. The twenty-mile trip included driving over the tallest bridge in the South at that time. I remember being terrified because I felt like I was blacking out, and I didn't understand what was happening to me. That's about all I remembered. Fortunately, I did get home safely. I don't know who spiked the punch, but I am still of the opinion that drinking is not for me.

I can't let my opinion keep me from using diluted vodka as an effective remedy, however, or from telling you about the amazing benefits of such use. But since we do have a real problem with alcohol abuse in this country, I want to make it clear that I do not recommend consuming alcohol or making it accessible to minors, etc. I will trust you to use good judgment.

Conclusion

There may never be a cure for the common cold, because it is not practical to make a vaccine for numerous viruses that can keep changing. On the other hand, having freedom from such misery is possible. We don't need vaccines for colds, because they can be stopped by using the simple hygiene steps outlined by Dr. Judd and modified by me.

There may never be a cure for respiratory allergies either. Who knows what pollen or other particle might be coming into our bodies next? Since we can easily stop the triggers, we don't need to be concerned with them. I can't promise that this will work for everybody, but you won't know unless you try it. I am always asking people to tell me if it doesn't work and, so far, no one has complained.

For those whose allergies are much worse than mine, I recommend that you learn to maximize your use of vitamins C and D before turning to more drastic treatments.

I have proven for myself, beyond any doubt, that avoidance of all congestion improves health. By stopping colds and allergic reactions, it goes without saying that we can avoid most of the secondary infections and chronic conditions that might follow.

I believe that some major changes need to come about in the way we pursue health and well-being. We know we can't keep killing the good microbes along with the bad. It is time to become more concerned about building and protecting our immunity, rather than trying to kill all germs.

We are learning more about what was discovered many years ago in regard to the potential of vitamin C to cure and prevent many diseases. We have recently discovered the benefits of maximizing our blood level of vitamin D. We cannot continue to allow these common-sense solutions to be restricted or denied. We should demand that simple treatments, such as an intravenous or intramuscular injection of vitamin C, be allowed in our hospitals for those who do not want to depend solely on pharmaceuticals.

The information age is moving faster than most of us grandmas. But I have reserved a domain name, http://www.howtostopcolds.com. My next project will be to build a website to keep you updated with any new information I might find on these subjects. I also plan to provide links to new products that become available for the remedies I have described.

In the meantime, I hope that sharing my discoveries will give you valuable insights that you can use to improve your health and help others.

Appendix A.1

Checklist—Colds & Allergies

Sore Throat: Gargle with 14% alcohol* to stop it quickly.

Sneezing, coughing, nasal congestion, sinus drip: Dip a cotton swab in 14% alcohol* and gently run it up the nostrils to kill viruses, bacteria, and even the histamine reaction.

Watering or irritated eyes: Put one drop of 14% alcohol* in an eye cup and fill with sterile water or saline eyewash.

Infection spreading into the lungs: Heat 4 teaspoons of 14% alcohol* just until steam starts coming up. Inhaling the vapor will destroy germs trying to invade the lungs.

Clearing the head: Inhale very warm salt water from the hand to the nose so that mucus is dissolved and removed from the nose, throat, sinuses, and back to the Eustachian tubes. (1/2 teaspoon of salt for each 8 oz. of sterile water)

Enhancing immunity: Add one teaspoon of ascorbic acid to a glass with one-half teaspoon of baking soda. Then add one inch of water. Let it fizz, add more water, and drink. Use good daily multivitamin supplements and take extra vitamin D3.

Earache: Pour several drops of 3% hydrogen peroxide into the ear. Let it bubble for a few minutes, then drain.

For complete instructions, see *How to Stop Colds, Allergies & More* by Carole S. Ramke.

* A mouth or nasal wash containing 14% alcohol (or 80-proof vodka, diluted with two parts of water)

Appendix A.2

Suggested Shopping List

Mouthwash (14% alcohol) or vodka

Salt: canning and pickling, kosher, or sea salt

Ascorbic acid powder and baking soda (or sodium ascorbate)

Empty bottles (3 oz.)

Cotton swabs

Hydrogen peroxide (3%)

Vitamin D3

Distilled or filtered water

Appendix B

Dilution of Alcohol, New Products

Dr. Judd recommended vodka, diluted to 14% alcohol. Vodka is plain ethanol or ethyl alcohol, which can be consumed by humans. Do not use other types of alcohol for this purpose.

Add two cups of distilled or filtered water to one cup of 80-proof vodka, to make a solution with 13.3% alcohol, which is probably close enough to 14%. I don't know if 14% is even necessary, or if that just happened to be the percentage in the mouthwash Dr. Judd used. I know it is definitely not necessary to use a solution stronger than 14% to get the desired results. You are in charge of determining what is best for you.

Since vodka is sold in different strengths (proof), here are my calculations for dilution to about 14% alcohol:

1 cup 80-proof vodka + 2 cups water = 13.3% alcohol

1 cup 90-proof vodka + 2 1/4 cups water = 13.9% alcohol

1 cup 100-proof vodka + 2 1/2 cups water = 14.3% alcohol

A half-pint of vodka (one cup) can be purchased for two or three dollars. Filtered or distilled water should be used for dilution to make an appropriate nasal wash. Your mixture can be stored in a one-quart canning jar or in some other suitable container with a child-proof cap if you have children. It should be labeled to show the contents, since it will look like water.

Along with the trial-sized personal products that are sold for travel use, you will usually find an assortment of little refill bottles which would be a more appropriate size to use with a small cotton swab. There might also be a bottle with a spray cap which you could adapt for use if you don't like to gargle. You could just spray your sore throat and spit into a tissue.

You might want to find an even smaller bottle to fill and keep in a sandwich bag with some cotton swabs. Then you will have convenient supplies to keep in your vehicle, desk, or bag. Don't forget to prevent access by children. I recently found a 1.5 ounce bottle of mouthwash with a child-proof cap. I will remove the label, refill it with my recipe of choice, and carry it in a small purse.

New Products

Shortly before sending this book to the printer, I discovered a mouthwash that is USDA certified organic. It contains only natural flavor, sweetener, and color—and none of the negative ingredients that are in conventional mouthwashes. I have ordered samples of several flavors so that I can try them before recommending. I will post my opinion on the website, as soon as it is up and running at http://www.howtostopcolds.com.

Appendix C.1

FOR IMMEDIATE RELEASE

Orthomolecular Medicine News Service, March 15, 2006

VITAMIN C HAS BEEN KNOWN TO FIGHT 30 MAJOR DISEASES...FOR OVER 50 YEARS

If so, why haven't you heard more about it? Why haven't more doctors used vitamin C as medicine?

Progress takes time. Fresh fruit was known to cure scurvy by 1753, yet governments ignored the fact for nearly 100 years. Countless thousands died in the meantime. The 19th century doctor who first advocated washing one's hands between patients died ignored and in disgrace with the medical profession. The toxic metal mercury was used as medicine into the twentieth century.

The first physician to aggressively use vitamin C to cure disease was Frederick R. Klenner, MD, beginning back in the early 1940's. Dr. Klenner successfully treated chicken pox, measles, mumps, tetanus and polio with huge doses of the vitamin.

The following is a complete list of the conditions that Dr. Klenner found that responded to extremely high dose vitamin C therapy:

Pneumonia

Encephalitis

Herpes Zoster (shingles)

Herpes Simplex

Mononucleosis

Pancreatitis

Hepatitis

Rocky Mountain Spotted Fever

Bladder Infection

Alcoholism

Arthritis

Some Cancers

Leukemia

Atherosclerosis

Ruptured Intervertebral Disc

High Cholesterol

Corneal Ulcer

Diabetes

Glaucoma

Schizophrenia

Burns and secondary infections

Heat Stroke

Radiation Burns

Heavy Metal Poisoning (Mercury, Lead)

Venomous Bites

Multiple Sclerosis

Chronic Fatigue

Complications of Surgery

This seems like an impossibly long list. At this point, one can either dismiss the subject or investigate further. Dr. Klenner chose to investigate. The result? He used massive doses of vitamin C for over forty years of family practice. He wrote two dozen medical papers on the subject. (1) It is difficult to ignore his success, but it has been done. Dr. Klenner wrote: "Some physicians would stand by and see their patient die rather than use ascorbic acid (vitamin C) because in their finite minds it exists only as a vitamin."

Vitamin C is remarkably safe even in enormously high doses. Compared to commonly used prescription drugs, side effects are virtually nonexistent. It does not cause kidney stones. In fact, vitamin C helps dissolve kidney stones and prevents their formation. William J. McCormick, MD, used vitamin C since the late 1940's to prevent and treat kidney stones. (2) Robert F. Cathcart III, MD, reports that he started using vitamin C in massive doses with patients in 1969. He writes: "I estimate that I have put 25,000 patients on massive doses of vitamin C and none have developed kidney stones." Said Dr. Klenner: "The ascorbic acid/kidney stone story is a myth." Recent scholarship has confirmed this. (4,5)

How much vitamin C is an effective therapeutic dose? Dr. Klenner administered up to an astounding 300,000 milligrams (mg) per day. Generally, he gave 350 to 700 mg per kilogram (2.2 lb) body weight per day. That is a lot of vitamin C.

But then again, look at that list of successes.

Dr. Klenner emphasized that small amounts do not work. He said, "If you want results, use adequate ascorbic acid."

For Further Reading:

The Vitamin C Connection, by Emanuel Cheraskin, MD et al (Harper and Row, 1983)

How To Live Longer and Feel Better, by Linus Pauling, PhD, (Freeman, 1986)

The Healing Factor: Vitamin C Against Disease, by Irwin Stone (Putnam, 1972) The complete text of this book is posted for free reading at http://vitamincfoundation.org/stone/ , a not-for-profit foundation's website.

Physicians and other health professionals may wish to read papers by William J. McCormick, MD, Linus Pauling, PhD, Abram Hoffer, MD, and Robert F. Cathcart III, MD.

References:

1. All of Dr. Klenner's papers are listed and summarized in the Clinical Guide to the Use of Vitamin C (ed. Lendon H. Smith, MD, Life Sciences Press, Tacoma, WA, 1988. This book is now posted in its entirety at http://www.seanet.com/~alexs/ascorbate/198x/smith-lh-clinical_guide_1988.htm, a non-commercial website.

2. McCormick WJ. Lithogenesis and hypovitaminosis. Medical Record 1946, 159:7, July.

4. Gerster H. No contribution of ascorbic acid to renal calcium oxalate stones. Ann Nutr Metab. 1997;41(5):269-82.

5. Hickey S and Roberts H. Vitamin C does not cause kidney stones. Orthomolecular Medicine News Service, July 5, 2005. http://orthomolecular.org/resources/omns/v01n07.shtml

Free Subscription Link: http://orthomolecular.org/subscribe.html

Archives: http://orthomolecular.org/resources/omns/index.shtml

Appendix C.2

FOR IMMEDIATE RELEASE

Orthomolecular Medicine News Service, December 8, 2009

VITAMIN C AND ACIDITY

What Form is Best?

(OMNS, December 8, 2009) Vitamin C is commonly taken in large quantities to improve health and prevent asthma, allergies, viral infection, and heart disease [1,2]. It is non-toxic and non-immunogenic, and does not irritate the stomach as drugs like aspirin can. Yet vitamin C (L-ascorbic acid) is acidic. So, a common question is, what are the effects from taking large quantities?

Ascorbic acid is a weak acid (pKa= 4.2) [3], only slightly stronger than vinegar. When dissolved in water, vitamin C is sour but less so than citric acid found in lemons and limes. Can large quantities of a weak acid such as ascorbate cause problems in the body? The answer is, sometimes, in some situations. However, with some simple precautions they can be avoided.

Acid in the Mouth

First of all, any acid can etch the surfaces of your teeth. This is the reason the dentist cleans your teeth and warns about plaque, for acid generated by bacteria in the mouth can etch your teeth to cause cavities. Cola soft drinks contain phosphoric acid, actually used by dentists to etch teeth before tooth sealants are applied. Like soft drinks, ascorbic acid will not cause etching of teeth if only briefly present. Often, vitamin C tablets are coated with a tableting ingredient such as magnesium stearate which prevents the ascorbate from dissolving immediately. Swallowing a vitamin C tablet without chewing it prevents its acid from harming tooth enamel.

Chewable Vitamin C Tablets

Chewables are popular because they taste sweet and so are good for encouraging children to take their vitamin C [4]. However, some chewable vitamin C tablets can contain sugar and ascorbic acid which, when chewed, is likely to stick in the crevices of your teeth. So, after chewing a vitamin C tablet, a good bit of advice is to rinse with water or brush your teeth. But the best way is to specifically select non-acidic vitamin C chewables, readily available in stores. Read the label to verify that the chewable is made entirely with non-acidic vitamin C.

Stomach Acidity

People with sensitive stomachs may report discomfort when large doses of vitamin C are taken at levels to prevent an acute viral infection (1,000-3,000 milligrams or more every 20 minutes) [1, 5]. In this case the ascorbic acid in the stomach can build up enough acidity to cause heartburn or a similar reaction. On the other hand, many people report no problems with acidity even when taking 20,000 mg in an hour. The acid normally present in the stomach, hydrochloric acid (HCl), is very strong: dozens of times more acidic than vitamin C. When one has swallowed a huge amount of ascorbate, the digestive tract is sucking it up into the bloodstream as fast as it can, but it may still take a while to do so. Some people report that they seem to sense ascorbic acid tablets "sitting" at the bottom of the stomach as they take time to dissolve. It is fairly easy to fix the problem by using buffered ascorbate, or taking ascorbic acid with food or liquids in a meal or snack. When the amount of vitamin C ingested is more than the gut can absorb, the ascorbate attracts water into the intestines creating a laxative effect. This saturation intake is called bowel tolerance. One should reduce the amount (by 20-50%) when this occurs [1].

Acid Balance in the Body

Does taking large quantities of an acid, even a weak acid like ascorbate, tip the body's acid balance (pH) causing health problems? No, because the body actively and constantly controls the pH of the bloodstream. The kidneys regulate the acid in the body over a long time period, hours to days, by selectively excreting either acid or basic components in urine. Over a shorter time period, minutes to hours, if the blood is too acid, the autonomic nervous system increases the rate of breathing, thereby removing more carbon dioxide from the blood, reducing its acidity. Some foods can indirectly cause acidity. For example, when more protein is eaten than necessary for maintenance and growth, it is metabolized into acid, which must be removed by the kidneys, generally as uric acid. In this case, calcium and/or magnesium are excreted along with the acid in the urine which can deplete our supplies of calcium and magnesium [6]. However, because ascorbic acid is a weak acid, we can tolerate a lot before it will much affect the body's acidity. Although there have been allegations about vitamin C supposedly causing kidney stones, there is no evidence for this, and its acidity and diuretic tendency actually tends to reduce kidney stones in most people who are prone to them [1,7]. Ascorbic acid dissolves calcium phosphate stones and dissolves struvite stones. Additionally, while vitamin C does increase oxalate excretion, vitamin C simultaneously inhibits the union of calcium and oxalate. [1,2].

Forms of Vitamin C

Ascorbate comes in many forms, each with a particular advantage. Ascorbic acid is the least expensive and can be purchased as tablets, timed release tablets, or powder. The larger tablets (1000-1500 mg) are convenient and relatively inexpensive. Timed-release tablets contain a long-chain carbohydrate which delays the stomach in dissolving the ascorbate, which is then released over a period of hours. This may have an advantage for maintaining a high level in the bloodstream. Ascorbic acid powder or crystals can be purchased in bulk relatively inexpensively. Pure powder is more quickly dissolved than tablets and therefore can be absorbed somewhat faster by the body. Linus Pauling favored taking pure ascorbic acid, as it is entirely free of tableting excipients.

Buffered Ascorbate

A fraction of a teaspoon of sodium bicarbonate (baking soda) has long been used as a safe and effective antacid which immediately lowers stomach acidity. When sodium bicarbonate is added to ascorbic acid, the bicarbonate fizzes (emitting carbon dioxide) which then releases the sodium to neutralize the acidity of the ascorbate.

Calcium ascorbate can be purchased as a powder and readily dissolves in water or juice. In this buffered form ascorbate is completely safe for the mouth and sensitive stomach and can be applied directly to the gums to help heal infections [8]. It is a little more expensive than the equivalent ascorbic acid and bicarbonate but more convenient. Calcium ascorbate has the advantage of being non-acidic. It has a slightly metallic taste and is astringent but not sour like ascorbic acid. 1000 mg of calcium ascorbate contains about 110 mg of calcium.

Other forms of buffered ascorbate include sodium ascorbate and magnesium ascorbate [9]. Most adults need 800—1200 mg of calcium and 400-600 mg of magnesium daily [6]. The label on the bottle of all these buffered ascorbates details how much "elemental" mineral is contained in a teaspoonful. They cost a little more than ascorbic acid.

Buffered forms of ascorbate are often better tolerated at higher doses than ascorbic acid, but they appear not to be as effective for preventing the acute symptoms of a cold. This may be because after they are absorbed they require absorbing an electron from the body to become effective as native ascorbate [1]. Some of types of vitamin C are proprietary formulas that claim benefits over standard vitamin C [9].

Liposomal Vitamin C

Recently a revolutionary form of ascorbate has become available. This form of vitamin C is packaged inside nano-scale phospholipid spheres ("liposomes"), much like a cell membrane protects its contents. The lipid spheres protect the vitamin C from degradation by the environment and are absorbed more quickly into the bloodstream. Liposomes are also known to facilitate intracellular uptake of their contents, which can cause an added clinical impact when delivering something such as vitamin C. This form is supposed to be 5-10 fold more absorbable than straight ascorbic acid. It is more expensive than ascorbic acid tablets or powder.

Ascorbyl Palmitate

Ascorbyl palmitate is composed of an ascorbate molecule bound to a palmitic acid molecule. It is amphipathic, meaning that it can dissolve in either water or fat, like the fatty acids in cell membranes. It is widely used as an antioxidant in processed foods, and used in topical creams where it is thought to be more stable than vitamin C. However, when ingested, the ascorbate component of ascorbyl palmitate is thought to be decomposed into the ascorbate and palmitic acid molecules so its special amphipathic quality is lost. It is also more expensive than ascorbic acid.

Natural Ascorbate

Natural forms of ascorbate derived from plants are available. Acerola, the "Barbados cherry," contains a large amount of vitamin C, depending on its ripeness, and was traditionally used to fight off colds. Tablets of vitamin C purified from acerola or rose hips are available but are generally low-dose and considerably more expensive than ascorbic acid. Although some people strongly advocate this type, Pauling and many others have stated that such naturally-derived vitamin C is no better than pure commercial ascorbate [2,9]. Bioflavonoids are antioxidants found in citrus fruits or rose hips and are thought to improve uptake and utilization of vitamin C. Generally, supplement tablets that contain bioflavonoids do not have enough to make much difference. For consumers on a budget, the best policy may be to buy vitamin C inexpensively whether or not it also contains bioflavonoids. Citrus fruits, peppers, and a number of other fruits and vegetables contain large quantities of bioflavonoids. This is one more reason to eat right as well as supplement.

References:

[1] Hickey S, Saul AW (2008) Vitamin C: The Real Story, the Remarkable and Controversial Healing Factor. ISBN-13: 9781591202233

[2] Pauling L (1986) How to Live Longer and Feel Better, by Linus Pauling (Revised version, 2006) ISBN-13: 9780870710964

[3] Handbook of Chemistry and Physics (2004), CRC Press, ISBN-13: 978-0849304859

[4] http://www.doctoryourself.com/megakid.html (Ideas on how to get children to take vitamin C.)

[5] Cathcart RF (1981) Vitamin C, titrating to bowel tolerance, anascorbemia, and acute induced scurvy. Med Hypotheses. 7:1359-1376.

[6] Dean C (2006) The Magnesium Miracle. (2006) ISBN-13: 9780345494580

[7] http://www.doctoryourself.com/kidney.html

[8] http://www.doctoryourself.com/gums.html (Healing gums with buffered ascorbate.)

See also: Riordan HD, Jackson, JA (1991) Topical ascorbate stops prolonged bleeding from tooth extraction. J Orthomolecular Med, 6:3-4, p 202. http://www.doctoryourself.com/news/v3n18.txt

[9] http://lpi.oregonstate.edu/infocenter/vitamins/vitaminC/vitCform.html(Information about different forms of vitamin C)

[10] http://www.doctoryourself.com/bioflavinoids.html

Free Subscription Link: http://orthomolecular.org/subscribe.html

Archives: http://orthomolecular.org/resources/omns/index.shtml

Appendix C.3

FOR IMMEDIATE RELEASE

Orthomolecular Medicine News Service, February 14, 2012

Vitamin C Prevents Vaccination Side Effects; Increases Effectiveness

by Thomas E Levy, MD, JD

(OMNS, Feb 14, 2012) The routine administration of vaccinations continues to be a subject of controversy in the United States, as well as throughout the world. Parents who want the best for their babies and children continue to be faced with decisions that they fear could harm their children if made incorrectly. The controversy over the potential harm of vaccinating, or of not vaccinating, will not be resolved to the satisfaction of all parties anytime soon, if ever. This brief report aims to offer some practical information to pediatricians and parents alike who want the best long-term health for their patients and children, regardless of their sentiments on the topic of vaccination in general.

While there seems to be a great deal of controversy over how frequently a vaccination might result in a negative outcome, there is little controversy that at least some of the time vaccines do cause damage. The question that then emerges is whether something can be done to minimize, if not eliminate, the infliction of such damage, however infrequently it may occur.

Causes of Vaccination Side Effects

When vaccines do have side effects and adverse reactions, these outcomes are often categorized as resulting from allergic reactions or the result of a negative interaction with compromised immune systems. While either of these types of reactions can be avoided subsequently when there is a history of a bad reaction having occurred at least once in the past as a result of a vaccination, it is vital to try to avoid encountering a negative outcome from occurring the first time vaccines are administered.

Due to the fact that all toxins, toxic effects, substantial allergic reactions, and induced immune compromise have the final common denominator of causing and/or resulting in the oxidation of vital biomolecules, the antioxidant vitamin C has proven to be the ultimate nonspecific antidote to whatever toxin or excess oxidative stress might be present. While there is also a great deal of dispute over the inherent toxicity of the antigens that many vaccines present to the immune systems of those vaccinated, there is no question, for example, that thimerosal, a mercury-containing preservative, is highly toxic when present in significant amounts. This then begs the question: Rather than argue whether there is an infinitesimal, minimal, moderate, or significant amount of toxicity associated with the amounts of thimerosal or other potentially toxic components presently being used in vaccines, why not just neutralize whatever toxicity is present as completely and definitively as possible?

Vitamin C is a Potent Antitoxin

In addition to its general antitoxin properties (Levy, 2002), vitamin C has been demonstrated to be highly effective in neutralizing the toxic nature of mercury in all of its chemical forms. In animal studies, vitamin C can prevent the death of animals given otherwise fatal doses of mercury chloride (Mokranjac and Petrovic, 1964). Having vitamin C on board prior to mercury exposure was able to prevent the kidney damage the mercury otherwise typically caused (Carroll et al., 1965). Vitamin C also blocked the fatal effect of mercury cyanide (Vauthey, 1951). Even the very highly toxic organic forms of mercury have been shown to be effectively detoxified by vitamin C (Gage, 1975).

Vitamin C Improves Vaccine Effectiveness

By potential toxicity considerations alone, then, there would seem to be no good reason not to pre- and post-medicate an infant or child with some amount of vitamin C to minimize or block the toxicity that might significantly affect a few. However, there is another compelling reason to make vitamin C an integral part of any vaccination protocol: Vitamin C has been documented to augment the antibody response of the immune system (Prinz et al., 1977; Vallance, 1977; Prinz et al., 1980; Feigen et al., 1982; Li and Lovell, 1985; Amakye-Anim et al., 2000; Wu et al., 2000; Lauridsen and Jensen, 2005; Azad et al., 2007). As the goal of any vaccination is to stimulate a maximal antibody response to the antigens of the vaccine while causing minimal to no toxic damage to the most sensitive of vaccine recipients, there would appear to be no medically sound reason not to make vitamin C a part of all vaccination protocols. Except in individuals with established, significant renal insufficiency, vitamin C is arguably the safest of all nutrients that can be given, especially in the amounts discussed below. Unlike virtually all prescription drugs and some supplements, vitamin C has never been found to have any dosage level above which it can be expected to demonstrate any toxicity.

Vitamin C Reduces Mortality in Vaccinated Infants and Children

Kalokerinos (1974) demonstrated repeatedly and quite conclusively that Aboriginal infants and children, a group with an unusually high death rate after vaccinations, were almost completely protected from this outcome by dosing them with vitamin C before and after vaccinations. The reason articulated for the high death rate was the exceptionally poor and near-scurvy-inducing (vitamin C-depleted) diet that was common in the Aboriginal culture. This also demonstrates that with the better nutrition in the United States and elsewhere in the world, the suggested doses of vitamin C should give an absolute protection against death (essentially a toxin-induced acute scurvy) and almost absolute protection against lesser toxic outcomes from any vaccinations administered. Certainly, there appears to be no logical reason not to give a nontoxic substance known to neutralize toxicity and stimulate antibody production, which is the whole point of vaccine administration.

Dosage Information for Pediatricians and Parents

Practically speaking, then, how should the pediatrician or parent proceed? For optimal antibody stimulation and toxin protection, it would be best to dose for three to five days before the shot(s) and to continue for at least two to three days following the shot. When dealing with infants and very young children, administering a 1,000 mg dose of liposome-encapsulated vitamin C would be both easiest and best, as the gel-like nature of this form of vitamin C allows a ready mixture into yogurt or any other palatable food, and the complete proximal absorption of the liposomes would avoid any possible loose stools or other possible undesirable bowel effects.

Vitamin C as sodium ascorbate powder will also work well. Infants under 10 pounds can take 500 mg daily in some fruit juice, while babies between 10 and 20 pounds could take anywhere from 500 mg to 1,000 mg total per day, in divided doses. Older children can take 1,000 mg daily per year of life (5,000 mg for a 5 year-old child, for example, in divided doses). If sodium must be avoided, calcium ascorbate is well-tolerated and, like sodium ascorbate, is non-acidic. Some but not all children's chewable vitamins are made with calcium ascorbate. Be sure to read the label. Giving vitamin C in divided doses, all through the day, improves absorption and improves tolerance. As children get older, they can more easily handle the ascorbic acid form of vitamin C, especially if given with meals. For any child showing significant bowel sensitivity, either use liposome-encapsulated vitamin C, or the amount of regular vitamin C can just be appropriately decreased to an easily tolerated amount.

Very similar considerations exist for older individuals receiving any of a number of vaccinations for preventing infection, such as the yearly flu shots. When there is really no urgency, and there rarely is, such individuals should supplement with vitamin C for several weeks before and several weeks after, if at all possible.

Even taking a one-time dose of vitamin C in the dosage range suggested above directly before the injections can still have a significant toxin-neutralizing and antibody-stimulating effect. It's just that an even better likelihood of having a positive outcome results from extending the pre- and post-dosing periods of time.

(Thomas Levy, MD, JD is a board-certified cardiologist and admitted to the bar in Colorado and the District of Colombia. He is the author of several books on vitamin C as well as numerous articles. By way of

disclaimer, he is a consultant to a company that sells a brand of liposome-encapsulated vitamin C. A vitamin C lecture by Dr. Levy may be viewed at: http://www.youtube.com/watch?v=k0GC9Fq8lfg)

References:

Amakye-Anim, J., T. Lin, P. Hester, et al. (2000) Ascorbic acid supplementation improved antibody response to infectious bursal disease vaccination in chickens. *Poultry Science* 79:680-688

Azad, I., J. Dayal, M. Poornima, and S. Ali (2007) Supra dietary levels of vitamins C and E enhance antibody production and immune memory in juvenile milkfish, *Chanos chanos* (Forsskal) to formalin-killed *Vibrio vulnificus. Fish & Shellfish Immunology* 23:154-163

Carroll, R., K. Kovacs, and E. Tapp (1965) Protection against mercuric chloride poisoning of the rat kidney. *Arzneimittelforschung* 15:1361-1363

Feigen, G., B. Smith, C. Dix, et al. (1982) Enhancement of antibody production and protection against systemic anaphylaxis by large doses of vitamin C. *Research Communications in Chemical Pathology and Pharmacology* 38:313-333

Gage, J. (1975) Mechanisms for the biodegradation of organic mercury compounds: the actions of ascorbate and of soluble proteins. *Toxicology and Applied Pharmacology* 32:225-238

Kalokerinos, A. (1974) *Every Second Child.* New Canaan, CT: Keats Publishing, Inc.

Lauridsen, C. and S. Jensen (2005) Influence of supplementation of all-rac-alpha-tocopheryl acetate preweaning and vitamin C postweaning on alpha-tocopherol and immune responses in piglets. *Journal of Animal Science* 83:1274-1286

Levy, T. (2004) *Curing the Incurable. Vitamin C, Infectious Diseases, and Toxins.* Henderson, NV: MedFox Publishing

Li, Y. and R. Lovell (1985) Elevated levels of dietary ascorbic acid increase immune responses in channel catfish. *The Journal of Nutrition* 115:123-131

Mokranjac, M. and C. Petrovic (1964) Vitamin C as an antidote in poisoning by fatal doses of mercury. *Comptes Rendus Hebdomadaires des Seances de l'Academie des Sciences* 258:1341-1342

Prinz, W., R. Bortz, B. Bregin, and M. Hersch (1977) The effect of ascorbic acid supplementation on some parameters of the human immunological defence system. *International Journal for Vitamin and Nutrition Research* 47:2248-257

Prinz, W., J. Bloch, G., G. Gilich, and G. Mitchell (1980) A systematic study of the effect of vitamin C supplementation on the humoral immune response in ascorbate-dependent mammals. I. The antibody response to sheep red blood cells (a T-dependent antigen) in guinea pigs. *International Journal for Vitamin and Nutrition Research* 50:294-300

Vallance, S. (1977) Relationships between ascorbic acid and serum proteins of the immune system. *British Medical Journal* 2:437-438

Vauthey, M. (1951) Protective effect of vitamin C against poisons. *Praxis (Bern)* 40:284-286

Wu, C., T. Dorairajan, and T. Lin (2000) Effect of ascorbic acid supplementation on the immune response of chickens vaccinated and challenged with infectious bursal disease virus. *Veterinary Immunology and Immunopathology* 74:145-152

Free Subscription Link: http://orthomolecular.org/subscribe.html

Archives: http://orthomolecular.org/resources/omns/index.shtml

Appendix C.4

FOR IMMEDIATE RELEASE

Orthomolecular Medicine News Service, May 14, 2012

Fukushima Radiation Release is Worse than You Have Been Told

What You Can Do to Protect Yourself

by Steve Hickey, PhD; Atsuo Yanagisawa, MD, PhD; Andrew W. Saul, PhD; Gert E. Schuitemaker, PhD; Damien Downing, MD

(OMNS May 14, 2012) People have been misinformed about the tragedy at Fukushima and its consequences. There is a continuing cover up, the reactors have not been stabilized, and radiation continues to be released. The Japanese College of Intravenous Therapy (JCIT) has recently released a video for people wishing to learn more about how to protect themselves from contamination by taking large doses of vitamin C.

Part 1 : http://www.youtube.com/watch?v=Rbm_MH3nSdM

Part 2 : http://www.youtube.com/watch?v=j4cyzts3lMo

Part 3 : http://www.youtube.com/watch?v=ZYiRo2Oucfo

Part 4 : http://www.youtube.com/watch?v=51le8FuuYJw

All four parts of the video are also available here http://firstlaw.wordpress.com/. Readers may link to, embed in their webpages, and make copies of the video for free distribution.

Japanese Government Minimizes Danger; Ignores Vitamin C

In the fall of 2011, JCIT presented a study that Fukushima workers had abnormal gene expression, which may be avoided using dietary antioxidants, especially vitamin C. The data was presented in Japan, Taiwan, and Korea. The JCIT sent letters to the government urging the government to tell the people how they may protect themselves from radiation. To date, the recommendation has been ignored by Japanese government and TEPCO (Tokyo Electric Power Company).

Linus Pauling gained the Nobel Peace Prize in part based on his calculations of the number of deaths from nuclear weapons fallout. [1] He was supported by physicist and father of the Soviet bomb Andrei Sakharov, who also later received the Nobel Prize for peace. [2] These and other scientists estimated that there would be an extra 10,000 deaths worldwide for each megaton nuclear test in the atmosphere. A nuclear reactor can contain much more radioactive material than a nuclear weapon. Fukushima had six reactors, plus stored additional radioactive material and nuclear waste.

How Radiation Damages Cells

Ionizing radiation acts to damage living tissue by forming free radicals. Essentially, electrons are ripped from molecules. Removing an electron from an atom or molecule turns it into an ion, hence the term ionizing radiation. X-rays, gamma rays, alpha- and beta-radiation are all ionizing.

Most of the damage occurs from ionizing radiation generating free radicals in water, as water molecules are by far the most abundant in the body. While avoiding unnecessary exposure to ionizing radiation is clearly preferable, people affected by Fukushima do not have the luxury of avoiding contamination.

Antioxidants: Free-Radical Scavengers

Free-radical scavengers, as the name suggests, mop up the damaging radicals produced by radiation. The more common term for free radical scavenger is antioxidant. Antioxidants replace the electrons stripped from molecules by ionizing radiation. Antioxidants have long been used in the treatment of radiation poisoning.[3-7] Most of the harm from ionizing radiation occurs from free radical damage which may be quenched by the free electrons antioxidants provide. Fortunately, safe antioxidants are widely available as nutritional supplements. Vitamin C is the prime example.

Why Vitamin C?

Vitamin C is of particular importance and should be included at high intakes for anyone trying to minimize radiation poisoning. High dose vitamin C provides continual antioxidant flow through the body. It is absorbed from the gut and helps to replenish the other antioxidants. When it is used up, it is excreted in the urine. Importantly, it can chelate, or grab onto, radioactive heavy metal atoms and help eliminate them from the body. Large dynamic flow doses of vitamin C (about 3,000 mg, taken 4 times a day for a total of 12,000 mg) would exemplify antioxidant treatment. Higher doses have been used by Dr. Atsuo Yanagisawa and colleagues. [8,9]

Shortly after the disaster, Dr. Damien Downing described how supplements can help protect against radioactive fallout.[10] OMNS issued an update on the response to Fukushima in Japan.[11] Recently, Dr. Gert Schuitemaker has provided a review of vitamin C as a radio-protectant for Fukushima contamination.[12]

Persons living in the areas affected by radioactive contamination can take antioxidant supplements, especially high doses of vitamin C, to counteract the negative consequences of long-term low dose radiation exposure, as well as to protect the health of coming generations.[12,13] People who have a possible internal or external radiation exposure should take antioxidant supplements to maintain an optimal antioxidant reserve. Because of the enormous size and oceanic spread of Fukushima contamination, this literally applies to everyone.

References:

1. The Nobel Foundation (1962) The Nobel Peace Prize 1962, Linus Pauling Biography, http://www.nobelprize.org/nobel_prizes/peace/laureates/1962/pauling-bio.html.

2. Sakharov A. (1975) The Nobel Peace Prize 1975, Andrei Sakharov, Autobiography, http://www.nobelprize.org/nobel_prizes/peace/laureates/1975/sakharov-autobio.html.

3. Brown SL, Kolozsvary A, Liu J, et al: Antioxidant diet supplementation starting 24 hours after exposure reduces radiation lethality. Radiat Res, 2010; 173: 462-468.

4. Zueva NA, Metelitsa LA, Kovalenko AN, et al: Immunomodulating effect of berlithione in clean-up workers of the Chernobyl nuclear plant accident [Article in Russian]. Lik Sprava, 2002; (1): 24-26.

5. Yamamoto T, Kinoshita M et al. Pretreatment with ascorbic acid prevents lethal gastrointestinal syndrome in mice receiving a massive amount of radiation. J Radiat Res (Tokyo) 2010; 51(2):145-56

6. Gaby A. Intravenous Nutrient Therapy: the "Myers' Cocktail". Alt Med Rev 2002; 7(5):389:403

7. Narra VR, Howell RW, Sastry KS, Rao DV. Vitamin C as a radioprotector against iodine-131 in vivo. J Nucl Med 1993; 34(4):637-40

8. Yanagisawa A. Orthomolecular approaches against radiation exposure. Presentation Orthomolecular Medicine Today Conference. Toronto 2011 http://www.doctoryourself.com/Radiation_VitC.pptx.pdf)

9. Green MH, Lowe JE et al. Effect of diet and vitamin C on DNA strand breakage in freshly-isolated human white blood cells. Mutat Res 1994; 316(2):91-102

10. Downing D. (2011) Radioactive Fallout: Can Nutritional Supplements Help?, A Personal Viewpoint, OMNS, May 10, http://www.orthomolecular.org/resources/omns/v07n04.shtml.

11. OMNS (2012) Vitamin C Prevents Radiation Damage, Nutritional Medicine in Japan, Orthomolecular Medicine News Service, February 1. http://orthomolecular.org/resources/omns/v08n06.shtml

12. Schuitemaker GE. Vitamin C as protection against radiation exposure. J Orthomolecular Med 2011, 26: 3; 141-145. [Also in Dutch: Schuitemaker G.E. Radioactiviteit in Japan: Orthomoleculair antwoord. Ortho 2011:3, June. http://www.ortho.nl]

13. Yanagisawa A, Uwabu M, Burkson BE, Weeks BS, Hunninghake R, Hickey S, Levy T, (2011) Environmental radioactivity and health. Official JCIT Statement, March 29. http://media.iv-therapy.jp/wp-content/uploads/2012/05/Statement.pdf

Free Subscription Link: http://orthomolecular.org/subscribe.html

Archives: http://orthomolecular.org/resources/omns/index.shtml

Appendix C.5

FOR IMMEDIATE RELEASE

Orthomolecular Medicine News Service, November 11, 2010

Vitamin C and The Law

A Personal Viewpoint by Thomas E. Levy, M.D., J.D.

(OMNS November 11, 2010) As a patient, you have the right to any therapy that is not prohibitively expensive, established to be effective, and not prohibitively toxic.

Any physician, or panel of hospital-based physicians, claiming that vitamin C is experimental, unapproved, and/or posing unwarranted risks to the health of the patient, is really only demonstrating a complete and total ignorance or denial of the scientific literature. A serious question as to what the real motivations might be in the withholding of such a therapy then arises.

A doctor has the right to refuse to see you or treat you. A doctor does not have the right to deny you any therapy that is inexpensive and known to be effective and nontoxic; if there is toxicity involved, the patient can discharge his responsibility for such toxicity with proper informed consent. A doctor does not have the right to deny you consultation with another doctor that may have conflicting medical points of view.

Just as ignorance of the law is no sound defense to legal charges brought against you, ignorance of medical fact is ultimately no sound defense for a doctor withholding valid treatment, especially when that information can be easily accessed.

While a hospital may or may not have a legal right to dictate to its physicians what they may or may not do, the patient and the family of the patient have the legal right to sue that hospital for any negative outcome that is perceived to directly result from such interference in patient care.

The patient and the family of the patient also have the right to sue any physician that refuses to administer an inexpensive, nontoxic therapy that is established to be of use in the medical literature, such as vitamin C, especially when no other options other than permitting the patient to die are offered. Doctors have a very strong herd mentality, and they do not thrive well when forced to deal with a lawsuit alone, and possibly not even with the backup of their malpractice insurance company, which would seriously question why an approved medicine such as vitamin C was withheld from the patient. Remember that any insurance company always looks for a legal way not to pay expenses or settlements.

In a court of law, legal decisions regarding medical issues are usually decided by comparing a doctor's actions (or inactions) to the accepted standards of medical practice in the community in question. The legal sticking points relate to how different that community might be from others, and whether the accepted standard of practice is too far deviated from overall mainstream medicine norms.

The legal system struggles with reconciling something well established in the medical literature, but not reflected in the standard medical textbooks. A case involving withheld vitamin C would not currently have any direct legal precedent of which I am aware, but there are multiple reasons to believe that the time is ripe for the law to rule for the patient's right to receive vitamin C in the hospital over the doctor's "right" to withhold it.

The time for changing the view of vitamin C by the law and mainstream medicine has arrived. Over the past 20 years, many more doctors have begun to routinely give 50 grams (50,000 mg) or more of vitamin C intravenously on a regular basis to patients with the entire gamut of medical conditions. These doctors have come from the same medical schools and postgraduate training programs as their unlike-minded mainstream counterparts, meaning they have the same traditional credentials and warrant equal consideration.

The law recognizes that there is no one perfect medical approach to a patient. Having an increasingly large body of doctors who recognize the importance of vitamin C will allow the courts to permit an additional "school of thought" as long as enough traditionally trained doctors think that way. The question yet to be legally determined is, How many such doctors is "enough?"

Under United States law, the long-standing *Frye* standard (1923) held that expert opinion based on a scientific technique is admissible only where the technique is generally accepted as reliable in the relevant scientific community. This standard made it almost impossible for any technique embraced by a minority, however competent or appropriately trained, to ever coexist with, much less supersede, a technique embraced by the larger scientific community. Basically, majority always wins, and minority always loses.

The *Daubert* standard (1993) finally replaced the *Frye* standard. *Daubert* held that the court should:

1. Evaluate whether the science can be or has been tested
2. Determine whether the science has been published or peer-reviewed
3. Consider the likelihood of error (quality and quantity of the data)
4. Evaluate the general acceptance of the theory in the scientific community

If the court is so inclined, the evaluation of general acceptance in the scientific (medical) community does not have to invoke the "majority rules" nature of the earlier *Frye* standard. Rather, it can allow the consideration that enough scientific studies embraced by enough qualified doctors could prevail legally. However, any final ruling would be heavily dependent on the particular facts of the case and the precise intervention requested of the court.

The principles of *Daubert* do not assure a victory for vitamin C proponents in a court of law, but they do allow an objective judge to see that the body of evidence supporting vitamin C usage is clearly established in the mainstream medical literature, warranting a thorough legal evaluation as to why it is not yet a permissible therapy. These principles allow for much more flexibility than the earlier *Frye* "majority rules" standard.

Also, with any individual case in which a doctor refuses to administer vitamin C and serious damage (including death) occurs, a strong legal case can now be made that the burden of proof falls with the doctor to show:

1. That the therapy was exceptionally expensive, toxic, and/or unproven
2. That the patient's best interests were somehow best served by withholding vitamin C

Always try to make an alliance with your doctor and avoid an adversarial relationship if at all possible. Theoretically, if your doctor really wants to do what is best for the patient and is not more concerned with being told what to do, much stress and conflict can be avoided by all. However, do not hesitate to let your doctor know directly that you will avail yourself of all your rights or your family member's rights as a patient to optimal health care if so forced.

A very common "out" in all of these scenarios is to suggest that "further studies" should be done. More information is always useful, but vitamin C has already been researched more than any other supplement, or even most pharmaceutical drugs, in the history of the planet. Don't allow another 70 years of research to transpire before its proper use begins.

Stand up for your rights today. The way medicine is practiced will never change until the public demands it and the law legitimizes it. Remember, it's your body and your health. Doctors are answerable to you, not you to them.

Thomas Edward Levy, M.D., J.D. is a graduate of the Tulane University School of Medicine and the University of Denver College of Law. He is board certified in Internal Medicine and is also a Fellow of the American College of Cardiology. He was admitted to the Colorado Bar in 1998 and the District of Columbia Bar in 1999. Dr. Levy is on the Editorial Board of the Orthomolecular Medicine News Service.

References:

Frye v. United States, 293 F. 1013 (D.C. Cir. 1923)

Daubert v. Merrell Dow Pharmaceuticals, 509 U.S. 579 (1993)

An expanded version of "Vitamin C and the Law" by Dr. Levy is available as a free pdf download at http://www.tomlevymd.com/downloads/VC.NZ.Sept.2010.pdf or http://www.doctoryourself.com/VC.NZ.Sept.2010.pdf

Free Subscription Link: http://orthomolecular.org/subscribe.html

Archives: http://orthomolecular.org/resources/omns/index.shtml

Appendix D.1

Professor Vieth and the Vitamin D Era

Posted on May 14, 2012 by John Cannell, MD

Historians will debate what started the vitamin D era, what paper triggered it, what scientists discovered its remarkable properties, what groups extolled it and what exactly changed people's mind from initially believing that vitamin D was toxic to believing it was healthy to take 5,000 IU/day. For me the question is easy. In the year 2001, I read a paper that changed my life. It was not even a new discovery or a new finding. Instead, it was a review paper written by Professor Reinhold Vieth of the University of Toronto and published in 1999. It is free to download in its entirety.

Vieth R. Vitamin D supplementation, 25-hydroxyvitamin D concentrations, and safety. Am J Clin Nutr. 1999 May;69(5):842-56.

I can remember reading it, thinking, rereading it, and thinking some more, perhaps as many as ten times. Professor Vieth filled the paper with well-established facts. For example, if you go out in the sun naked in the summer around noon and turn slightly pink, you make as much as 20,000 IU of vitamin D.

Those facts led me to the simple question of "Why." Why so much so fast? Why would nature make such a system that made so much so fast? I thought and thought and read and read and the only answer I could come up with was, "Probably for a good reason." That's not much of an answer in light of what we know today, but it was good enough to start the Vitamin D Council, and it was good enough to realize that my life's work was to spread the word. With sickness in the pit of my stomach, I feared that modern medicine had made a terrible mistake in labeling vitamin D toxic, and thus severely limiting the amount in foods and supplements. I also realized that when science makes a great error, great good is waiting around the corner, if someone can correct that error.

Almost every day the answer, "probably for a good reason," sounds dumber and dumber. We are rapidly finding out the real answers. Every day another scientist publishes a study showing benefits from everything from pediatric cardiomyopathy (infantile heart failure) to hepatitis C to asthma. Nature gives humans such doses of vitamin D from the sun because vitamin D is the only known building block of a potent substance that functions as the "repair and maintenance" steroid hormone of the human body.

However, Vieth's paper did something else: it convincingly argued that our fear of vitamin D toxicity verged on hysteria and had nothing to do with science. He meticulously researched all the old publications that claimed vitamin D was toxic only to discover a house of cards, papers that referred back to each other and not to any actual scientific papers showing toxicity. That is, he elegantly exposed that 10,000 IU/day could not be toxic (not if we make that much and more from the sun) and that toxicity more likely starts somewhere well above 20,000 IU/day.

About John Cannell, MD

Dr. John Cannell is founder of the Vitamin D Council. He has written many peer-reviewed papers on vitamin D and speaks frequently across the United States on the subject. Dr. Cannell holds an M.D. and has served the medical field as a general practitioner, itinerant emergency physician, and psychiatrist.

Appendix D.2

News Release

November 30, 2010

Today the Food and Nutrition Board has Failed Millions

After 13 years of silence, the quasi-governmental agency, the Institute of Medicine's (IOM) Food and Nutrition Board (FNB), yesterday recommended that a three-pound premature infant can take virtually the same amount of vitamin D as a 300 pound pregnant woman. While that 400 IU/day dose is close to adequate for infants, 600 IU/day in pregnant women will do nothing to help the three childhood epidemics most closely associated with gestational and early childhood vitamin D deficiencies: asthma, auto-immune disorders, and, as recently reported in the largest pediatric journal in the world, autism (1). Professor Bruce Hollis of the Medical University of South Carolina has shown pregnant and lactating women need at least 5,000 IU/day, not 600.

The FNB also reported that vitamin D toxicity might occur at an intake of 10,000 IU/day (250 micrograms), although they could produce no reproducible evidence that 10,000 IU/day has ever caused toxicity in humans and only one poorly conducted study indicating 20,000 IU/day may cause mild elevations in serum calcium but not clinical toxicity.

Viewed with different measure, this FNB report recommends that an infant should take 10 micrograms/day (400 IU) and the pregnant women 15 micrograms/day (600 IU). As a single 30 minutes dose of summer sunshine gives adults more than 10,000 IU (250 micrograms), the FNB is apparently also warning that natural vitamin D input—as occurred from the sun before the widespread use of sunscreen—is dangerous. That is, the FNB is implying that God does not know what she is doing.

Disturbingly, this FNB committee focused on bone health, just like they did 14 years ago. They ignored the thousands of studies from the last ten years that showed higher doses of vitamin D helps: heart health, brain health, breast health, prostate health, pancreatic health, muscle health, nerve health, eye health, immune health, colon health, liver health, mood health, skin health, and especially fetal health. Tens of millions of pregnant women and their breastfeeding infants are severely vitamin D deficient, resulting in a great increase in the medieval disease, rickets. The FNB report seems to reason that if so many pregnant women have low vitamin D blood levels then it must be OK because such low levels are so common. However, such circular logic simply represents the cave man existence of most modern day pregnant women.

Hence, if you want to optimize your vitamin D levels—not just optimize the bone effect—supplementing is crucial. But it is almost impossible to significantly raise your vitamin D levels when supplementing at only 600 IU/day (15 micrograms). Pregnant women taking 400 IU/day have the same blood levels as pregnant women not taking vitamin D; that is, 400 IU is a meaninglessly small dose for pregnant women. Even taking 2,000 IU/day of vitamin D will only increase the vitamin D levels of most pregnant women by about 10 points, depending mainly on their weight. Professor Bruce Hollis has shown that 2,000 IU/day does not raise vitamin D to healthy or natural levels in either pregnant or lactating women. Therefore supplementing with higher amounts—like 5000 IU/day—is crucial for those women who want their fetus to enjoy optimal vitamin D levels, and the future health benefits that go along with it.

For example, taking only two of the hundreds of recently published studies, Professor Urashima and colleagues in Japan gave 1,200 IU/day of vitamin D3 for six months to Japanese 10 year-olds in a randomized controlled trial. They found vitamin D dramatically reduced the incidence of influenza A as well as the episodes of asthma attacks in the treated kids while the placebo group was not so fortunate. If Dr. Urashima had followed the newest FNB recommendations, it is unlikely that 400 IU/day treatment arm would have done much of anything and some of the treated young teenagers may have come to serious harm without the vitamin D. Likewise, a randomized controlled prevention trial of adults by Professor Joan Lappe and colleagues at Creighton University, which showed dramatic improvements in the health of internal organs, used more than twice the FNB's new adult recommendations.

Finally, the FNB committee consulted with 14 vitamin D experts and—after reading these 14 different reports—the FNB decided to suppress their reports. Many of these 14 consultants are either famous vitamin D researchers, like Professor Robert Heaney at Creighton, or in the case of Professor Walter Willett at Harvard, the single best-known nutritionist in the world. So, the FNB will not tell us what Professors Heaney and Willett thought of their new report? Why not? Yesterday, the Vitamin D Council directed our attorney to file a federal Freedom of Information (FOI) request to the IOM's FNB for the release of these 14 reports.

I, my family, most of my friends, hundreds of patients, and thousands of readers of the Vitamin D Council newsletter, have been taking 5,000 IU/day for up to eight years. Not only have they reported no significant side-effects, indeed, they have reported greatly improved health in multiple organ systems. My advice: especially for pregnant women, continue taking 5,000 IU/day until your (OH) D] is between 50 ng/ml and 80 ng/ml (the vitamin D blood levels obtained by humans who live and work in the sun and the midpoint of the current reference ranges at all American laboratories). Gestational vitamin D deficiency is not only associated with rickets, but a significantly increased risk of neonatal pneumonia (2), a doubled risk for preeclampsia (3), a tripled risk for gestational diabetes (4), and a quadrupled risk for primary cesarean section (5).

Yesterday, the FNB failed millions of pregnant women whose as yet unborn babies will pay the price. Let us hope the FNB will comply with the spirit of "transparency" by quickly responding to our Freedom of Information requests.

John Cannell, MD

The Vitamin D Council
1241 Johnson Avenue, #134
San Luis Obispo, CA 93401

(1) Cannell JJ.. On the aetiology of autism. Acta Paediatr. 2010 Aug;99(8):1128-30. Epub 2010 May 19.
(2)Karatekin G, Kaya A, Salihoglu O, Balci H, Nuhoglu A. Association of subclinical vitamin D deficiency in newborns with acute lower respiratory infection and their mothers. Eur J Clin Nutr. 2009;63(4):473-7.
(3) Bodnar LM, Catov JM, Simhan HN, Holick MF, Powers RW, Roberts JM. Maternal vitamin D deficiency increases the risk of preeclampsia. J Clin Endocrinol Metab. 2007;92(9):3517-22.
(4) Zhang C, Qiu C, Hu FB, David RM, van Dam RM, Bralley A, Williams MA. Maternal Plasma 25-hydroxyvitamin D Concentrations and the Risk for Gestational Diabetes Mellitus. PLoS One. 2008;3(11):e3753.
(5) Merewood A, Mehta SD, Chen TC, Bauchner H, Holick MF. Association Between Vitamin D Deficiency and Primary Cesarean Section. J Clin Endocrinol Metab. 2009;94(3):940-5.

Follow-up: The chairperson of the committee of the Institute of Medicine's (IOM) Food and Nutrition Board (FNB) claimed immunity to the Freedom of Information Request.

Appendix D.3

News Release

Date: February 22, 2011

Higher Vitamin D Intake Needed to Reduce Cancer Risk

Researchers at the University of California, San Diego School of Medicine and Creighton University School of Medicine in Omaha have reported that markedly higher intake of vitamin D is needed to reach blood levels that can prevent or markedly cut the incidence of breast cancer and several other major diseases than had been originally thought. The findings are published February 21 in the journal *Anticancer Research.*

While these levels are higher than traditional intakes, they are largely in a range deemed safe for daily use in a December 2010 report from the National Academy of Sciences Institute of Medicine.

"We found that daily intakes of vitamin D by adults in the range of 4000-8000 IU are needed to maintain blood levels of vitamin D metabolites in the range needed to reduce by about half the risk of several diseases—breast cancer, colon cancer, multiple sclerosis, and type 1 diabetes," said Cedric Garland, DrPH, professor of family and preventive medicine at UC San Diego Moores Cancer Center. "I was surprised to find that the intakes required to maintain vitamin D status for disease prevention were so high—much higher than the minimal intake of vitamin D of 400 IU/day that was needed to defeat rickets in the 20th century."

"I was not surprised by this" said Robert P. Heaney, MD, of Creighton University, a distinguished biomedical scientist who has studied vitamin D need for several decades. "This result was what our dose-response studies predicted, but it took a study such as this, of people leading their everyday lives, to confirm it."

The study reports on a survey of several thousand volunteers who were taking vitamin D supplements in the dosage range from 1000 to 10,000 IU/day. Blood studies were conducted to determine the level of 25-vitamin D—the form in which almost all vitamin D circulates in the blood.

"Most scientists who are actively working with vitamin D now believe that 40 to 60 ng/ml is the appropriate target concentration of 25-vitamin D in the blood for preventing the major vitamin D-deficiency related diseases, and have joined in a letter on this topic," said Garland. "Unfortunately, according to a recent National Health and Nutrition Examination Survey, only 10 percent of the US population has levels in this range, mainly people who work outdoors."

Interest in larger doses was spurred in December of last year, when a National Academy of Sciences Institute of Medicine committee identified 4000 IU/day of vitamin D as safe for everyday use by adults and children nine years and older, with intakes in the range of 1000-3000 IU/day for infants and children through age eight years old.

While the IOM committee states that 4000 IU/day is a safe dosage, the recommended minimum daily intake is only 600 IU/day.

"Now that the results of this study are in, it will become common for almost every adult to take 4000 IU/day," Garland said. "This is comfortably under the 10,000 IU/day that the IOM Committee Report considers as the lower limit of risk, and the benefits are substantial." He added that people who may have contraindications should discuss their vitamin D needs with their family doctor.

"Now is the time for virtually everyone to take more vitamin D to help prevent some major types of cancer, several other serious illnesses, and fractures," said Heaney.

Other co-authors of the article were Leo Baggerly, PhD, and Christine French.

More facts are available from Anticancer Research: www.GrassrootsHealth.net; and the National Academy of Sciences—Institute of Medicine:

http://www.iiar-anticancer.org/openAR/journals/index/php/anticancer/article/view/215

Reprinted with permission:

Kim Edwards, Sr. Public Information Officer
University of California, San Diego Health Sciences
200 West Arbor Drive #8907
San Diego, California 92103-8907

Appendix D.4

Proceed at Your Peril

Posted on May 21, 2012 by John Cannell, MD

It's becoming increasingly clear that strict avoidance of ultraviolet (UV) light significantly increases the risk of dying from internal cancers. Yes, the risks of developing one of the major cancer killers increase when we avoid the sun. In fact, Dr. Tuohimaa and company recently showed that the risk of developing almost all varieties of fatal internal cancers is less in those who spend time in the sun.

Apparently, none of the organizations and government agencies with "avoid the sun" campaigns considered the possibility that avoiding the sun would harm anyone. Seemingly, no one thought about how UV light might help us. No one remembered that humans evolved in the sun, living naked in the sun for almost all of our two million years on the planet. Only in recent years did we start avoiding the sun. In other words, we started messing with Mother Nature.

Furthermore, when the government and medical organizations began to tell us to avoid the sun in the early 1980s, they literally forgot to tell us to take a vitamin D supplement to make up for the vitamin D we'd no longer be making via the sun. Since so much vitamin D is made by the sun, you'd think the experts would have said, "Oh yes, be sure to take a vitamin D supplement if you avoid the sun." Neither medical organizations nor the government did so.

Before you decide to just take a vitamin D supplement and completely avoid the UV light, think about a Greek word. It's "hubris," which means overbearing pride, presumption, or arrogance. If you decide simply to take a pill while completely avoiding all UV light, you are arrogantly assuming that modern science understands all of the beneficial effects of UV light and that the only good that UV light does is make vitamin D. You take pride that science is complete and knows everything. The Greeks abhorred such hubris and believed that the gods often punished it.

Let me give you an example. Multiple sclerosis (MS) is a terrible disease. Dr. Becklund and Professor Hector Deluca of the University of Wisconsin were the first to discover that vitamin D retarded progression of an animal model of MS called "experimental autoimmune encephalomyelitis" (EAE). While vitamin D suppresses the progression of EAE, continuous treatment with artificial ultraviolet radiation (as in sunbeds) works even better. He concluded that ultraviolet light was likely suppressing EAE independent of vitamin D production, and that vitamin D supplementation alone cannot replace UV light in an animal model of MS. If true in humans, it means that UV light contains something good in addition to vitamin D.

The wisest course is to get safe, short, reasonable, and regular full-body exposures during the warm months and judiciously use low-pressure UV beds and vitamin D supplements in the winter, recognizing that scientists and doctors don't know everything. In fact, they got us into this vitamin D deficiency epidemic in the first place. Keep in mind that your ancestors evolved naked on the savannahs of equatorial Africa, eating bugs and roots from the ground with the sun shining directly overhead. Humans have a long evolutionary bond with the sun. When, with hubris, you sever the relationship between yourself and UV light, proceed at your peril.

Sources:

Becklund BR, Severson KS, Vang SV, DeLuca HF. UV radiation suppresses experimental autoimmune encephalomyelitis independent of vitamin D production. Proc Natl Acad Sci U S A. 2010 Apr 6;107(14):6418-23. Epub 2010 Mar 22.

Kricker A, Armstrong B. Does sunlight have a beneficial influence on certain cancers? Prog Biophys Mol Biol. 2006 Sep;92(1):132-9. Epub 2006 Feb 28.

Tuohimaa P, et al. Does solar exposure, as indicated by the non-melanoma skin cancers, protect from solid cancers: vitamin D as a possible explanation. Eur J Cancer. 2007 Jul;43(11):1701-12. Epub 2007 May 30.

van der Rhee HJ, de Vries E, Coebergh JW. Does sunlight prevent cancer? A systematic review. Eur J Cancer. 2006 Sep;42(14):2222-32. Epub 2006 Aug 10

About John Cannell, MD

Dr. John Cannell is founder of the Vitamin D Council. He has written many peer-reviewed papers on vitamin D and speaks frequently across the United States on the subject. Dr. Cannell holds an M.D. and has served the medical field as a general practitioner, itinerant emergency physician, and psychiatrist.

Appendix D.5

Vitamin D, UV Exposure, and Skin Cancer in a Nutshell

Posted on May 22, 2012, by Brant Cebulla

May 25th is National Don't Fry Day, a campaign by the National Council for Skin Cancer Prevention to make sure people protect themselves from the sun. They contend that skin cancer is a growing epidemic so be sure to protect yourself from the sun, which doesn't make perfect sense considering skin cancer is increasing despite the growing trend to stay out of the sun.

Nevertheless, it's a good week to take a look at what is known about vitamin D, UV and sun exposure, and skin cancer, especially heading into Memorial Day Weekend and the beginning of summer. We're here to break it down for you!

To date, research is not complete and there are many unknowns. Generally speaking, UV exposure is a risk factor for skin cancer. On the other hand, vitamin D sufficiency is protective against skin cancer. You can see the contradiction here, but let's take a closer look.

There are three types of skin cancer:

1. Basal cell carcinoma: The role of UV exposure in basal cell carcinoma (BCC) is not clear, but observational studies have found a 50% increased risk in those who tan. The number of BCC cases outnumbers the number of squamous cell carcinoma cases (SCC) by a ratio of 4 to 1, and approximately 3 in 10 people will develop it in their lifetime. In a randomized controlled trial, the use of sunscreen did not reduce the risk of developing BCC, which makes the relationship between UV exposure and BCC a bit puzzling.

2. Squamous cell carcinoma: The risk of SCC is more strongly related to cumulative UV exposure. Observational studies have found a two-fold increased risk in those who tan. In the same randomized controlled trial with BCC, researchers found a 40% reduction in the risk of SCC with use of sunscreen.

3. Malignant melanoma: The incidence of stage one melanoma has increased since the 1950s, though some studies suggest this rise can be attributed to increased diagnosis and not incidence. It is generally accepted that melanoma risk is determined by a combination of genetic factors and UV exposure. The greatest risk factor is the number of moles one is born with, and it is thought, though yet to be proven, that UV exposure induces these types of moles to become malignant.

Paradoxically, sun exposure and UVB increase vitamin D levels, a known anti-cancer agent. Although there have been no controlled trials that look at vitamin D for prevention or treatment of skin cancers, researchers have identified mechanisms where vitamin D inhibits all three types of skin cancer, and they have demonstrated this in animal models.

Furthermore, an observational study found that vitamin D levels greater than 30 ng/ml decreased the incidence of non-melanoma skin cancers by half compared to those with levels under 16 ng/ml. Levels between 16 to 30 ng/ml were not quite as protective as levels above 30 ng/ml.

To add to the confusion, one study found no correlation between vitamin D levels and skin cancer risk, while another found a correlation between higher levels of vitamin D and higher incidence of non-melanoma skin cancers, probably due to overly excessive sun exposure.

What does this all mean? That there is probably a sweet spot for sun exposure. You need sun exposure to produce vitamin D, but you don't want to overexpose yourself. Get some sun exposure for vitamin D production, but don't burn yourself.

Given all this, the Vitamin D Council recommends these 6 essential points regarding your sun exposure habits:

1. Regular and sensible sun exposure is a healthy practice. Vitamin D production is very high when your shadow is shorter than you are.

2. When sunbathing, the Vitamin D Council recommends exposing your skin for half the time it takes to turn pink. After this, cover up with clothing or shade.

3. Overexposure is unnecessary and dangerous.

4. If the intention in sunbathing is to produce vitamin D, the Vitamin D Council does not recommend sunscreen as it will not allow you to optimally produce vitamin D. Furthermore, sunscreen is not proven to be consistently protective and safe.

5. Tanning beds with low pressure lamps are a suitable substitute to sun exposure as long as the same sensibility is applied to their use. Don't burn! Just get a little vitamin D.

6. Consistent sun exposure in the 21st century is not easily achieved. Additional measures should be taken, including supplementation and/or the use of low pressure tanning beds.

Let's also not forget that vitamin D does lots of things, and that skin cancer is a small part of the equation. One million people die per year due to breast and colon cancers; cancers where vitamin D deficiency is a known risk factor. Without reducing the seriousness of melanoma (which accounts for fifty thousand deaths worldwide per year), common sense suggests that the benefits of sensible sun exposure are well worth the risk.

Sources:

Tang, JY and Epstein Jr, EH. Vitamin D and Skin Cancer. In Vitamin D, Third Edition by Feldman D, Pike JW, and Adams JS. Elsevier Academic Press, 2011.

About Brant Cebulla

Brant Cebulla is the Development Director for the Vitamin D Council. He believes Paleo dieting, high intensity fitness and sun exposure are the future in nutrition.

Appendix E

FOR IMMEDIATE RELEASE

Orthomolecular Medicine News Service, October 14, 2011

Vitamin E Attacked Again

Of Course. Because It Works.

by Andrew W. Saul

Editor, Orthomolecular Medicine News Service

(OMNS, Oct 14, 2011) The very first Orthomolecular Medicine News Service release was on the clinical benefits of vitamin E. That was seven years ago. (1) In fact, the battle over vitamin E has been going full-tilt for over 60 years. (2)

Well, you can say one thing for vitamin critics: at least they are consistent. Consistently wrong, but consistent.

A recent accusation against vitamin E is that somehow it increases risk of prostate cancer. (3) That is nonsense. If you take close look at the numbers, you will see that "Compared with placebo, the absolute increase in risk of prostate cancer per 1000 person-years was 1.6 for vitamin E, 0.8 for selenium, and 0.4 for the combination." That works out to be a claimed 0.63% increase risk with vitamin E alone, 0.24% increase in risk with vitamin E and selenium, and 0.15% increase in risk for selenium alone.

Note the decimal points: these are very small figures. But more importantly, note that the combination of selenium with vitamin E resulted in a much smaller number of deaths. If vitamin E were really the problem, vitamin E with selenium would have been a worse problem. Selenium recharges vitamin E, recycling it and effectively rendering it more potent. Something is wrong here, and it isn't the vitamin E. Indeed, a higher dose of vitamin E might work as well as E with selenium, and be more protective.

And, in fact, this study did show that supplementation was beneficial. Vitamin E and selenium reduced risk of all-cause mortality by about 0.2%., and also reduced the risk of serious cardiovascular events by 0.3%. Vitamin E reduced risk of serious cardiovascular events by 0.7%. But what you were told, and just about all you were told, was "Vitamin E causes cancer!"

The oldest political trick in the book is to create doubt, then fear, and then conformity of action. The pharmaceutical industry knows this full well. One does not waste time and money attacking something that does not work. Vitamin E works, and the evidence is abundant.

Specifically in regards to prostate cancer, new research published in the *International Journal of Cancer* has shown that **gamma-tocotrienol, a cofactor found in natural vitamin E preparations, actually kills prostate cancer stem cells.** (4) As you would expect, these are the very cells from which prostate cancer develops. They are or quickly become chemotherapy-resistant. And yet natural vitamin E complex contains the very thing to kill them. Mice given gamma-tocotrienol orally had an astonishing 75% decrease in tumor formation. Gamma-tocotrienol also is effective against existing prostate tumors. (5,6)

Additionally:

- **Vitamin E reduces mortality by 24% in persons 71 or older.** Even persons who smoke live longer if they take vitamin E. Hemila H, Kaprio J. Age Ageing, 2011. 40(2): 215-220. January 17. http://ageing.oxfordjournals.org/content/40/2/215.short
- **Taking 300 IU vitamin E per day reduces lung cancer by 61%.** (Mahabir S, Schendel K, Dong YQ et al. Dietary alpha-, beta-, gamma- and delta-tocopherols in lung cancer risk. Int J Cancer. 2008 Sep 1;123(5):1173-80.) http://www.ncbi.nlm.nih.gov/pubmed/18546288 For further information: Vitamin E prevents lung cancer. Orthomolecular Medicine News Service, Oct 29, 2008. http://orthomolecular.org/resources/omns/v04n18.shtml

- **Vitamin E is an effective treatment for atherosclerosis.** Drs. Wilfrid and Evan Shute knew this half a century ago. (1) In 1995, JAMA published research that confirmed it, saying: "Subjects with supplementary vitamin E intake of 100 IU per day or greater demonstrated less coronary artery lesion progression than did subjects with supplementary vitamin E intake less than 100 IU per day." (Hodis HN, Mack WJ, LaBree L et al. Serial coronary angiographic evidence that antioxidant vitamin intake reduces progression of coronary artery atherosclerosis. JAMA, 1995. 273:1849-1854.) http://jama.ama-assn.org/content/273/23/1849.short
- **400 to 800 IU of vitamin E daily reduces risk of heart attack by 77%.** (Stephens NG et al. Randomized controlled trial of vitamin E in patients with coronary artery disease: Cambridge Heart Antioxidant Study (CHAOS). Lancet, March 23, 1996; 347:781-786.) http://www.ncbi.nlm.nih.gov/pubmed/8622332
- **Increasing vitamin E with supplements prevents COPD** [Chronic obstructive pulmonary disease, emphysema, chronic bronchitis] (Agler AH et al. Randomized vitamin E supplementation and risk of chronic lung disease (CLD) in the Women's Health Study. American Thoracic Society 2010 International Conference, May 18, 2010.) Summary at http://www.thoracic.org/media/press-releases/conference/articles/2010/vitamine-e.pdf
- **800 IU vitamin E per day is a successful treatment for fatty liver disease.** (Sanyal AJ, Chalasani N, Kowdley KV et al. Pioglitazone, vitamin E, or placebo for nonalcoholic steatohepatitis. N Engl J Med. 2010 May 6;362(18):1675-85.) http://www.ncbi.nlm.nih.gov/pubmed/20427778
- **Alzheimer's patients who take 2,000 IU of vitamin E per day live longer.** (Pavlik VN, Doody RS, Rountree SD, Darby EJ. Vitamin E use is associated with improved survival in an Alzheimer's disease cohort. Dement Geriatr Cogn Disord. 2009;28(6):536-40.) Summary at http://www.associated

content.com/article/719537/alzheimers_patients_who_take_vitamin.html?cat=5

See also: Grundman M. Vitamin E and Alzheimer disease: the basis for additional clinical trials. Am J Clin Nutr. 2000 Feb;71(2):630S-636S. Free access to full text at http://www.ajcn.org/cgi/content/full/71/2/630s)

- **400 IU of vitamin E per day reduces epileptic seizures in children by more than 60%.** (Ogunmekan AO, Hwang PA. A randomized, double-blind, placebo-controlled, clinical trial of D-alpha-tocopheryl acetate [vitamin E], as add-on therapy, for epilepsy in children. Epilepsia. 1989 Jan-Feb; 30(1):84-9.) http://www.ncbi.nlm.nih.gov/pubmed/2643513
- **Vitamin E supplements help prevent amyotrophic lateral sclerosis (ALS).** This important finding is the result of a 10-year-plus Harvard study of over a million persons. (Wang H, O'Reilly EJ, Weisskopf MG, et al. Vitamin E intake and risk of amyotrophic lateral sclerosis: a pooled analysis of data from 5 prospective cohort studies. Am. J. Epidemiol, 2011. 173 (6): 595-602. March 15) http://aje.oxfordjournals.org/content/173/6/595.short
- **Vitamin E is more effective than a prescription drug in treating chronic liver disease** (nonalcoholic steatohepatitis). Said the authors: "The good news is that this study showed that cheap and readily available vitamin E can help many of those with this condition." Sanyal AJ, Chalasani N, Kowdley KV et al. Pioglitazone, vitamin E, or placebo for nonalcoholic steatohepatitis. N Engl J Med. 2010 May 6;362(18):1675-85. http://www.nejm.org/doi/full/10.1056/NEJMoa0907929

What Kind of Vitamin E?

Which work best: natural or synthetic vitamins? The general debate might not end anytime soon. However, with vitamin E, we already know. The best E is the most natural form, generally called "mixed natural tocopherols and tocotrienols." This is very different from the synthetic form, DL-alpha tocopherol. In choosing a vitamin E supplement, you should carefully read the label…the entire label. It is remarkable how many natural-looking brown bottles with natural-sounding brand names contain a synthetic vitamin. And no, we do not make brand recommendations. Furthermore, OMNS has no commercial affiliations or funding.

Unfortunately, that's not the case with some authors of the negative vitamin E paper. (3) You will not see this in the abstract at the JAMA website, of course, but if you read the entire paper, and get to the very last page (1556), you'll find the "Conflict of Interest" section. Here you will discover that a number of the study authors have received money from pharmaceutical companies, including Merck, Pfizer, Sanofi-Aventis, AstraZeneca, Abbott, GlaxoSmith-Kline, Janssen, Amgen, Firmagon, and Novartis. In terms of cash, these are some of the largest corporations on the planet.

Well how about that: a "vitamins are dangerous" article, in one of the most popular medical journals, with lots of media hype…and the pharmaceutical industry's fingerprints all over it.

So How Much Vitamin E?

More than the RDA, and that's for certain. A common dosage range for vitamin E is between 200 and 800 IU/day. Some orthomolecular physicians advocate substantially more than that. The studies cited above will give you a ballpark idea. However, this is an individual matter for you and your practitioner to work out. Your own reading and research, before you go to your doctor, will help you determine optimal intake. If your doctor quotes a negative vitamin study, then haul out the positive ones. You may start with this article. There are more links to more information at http://orthomolecular.org/resources/omns/v06n09.shtml and http://orthomolecular.org/resources/omns/v06n25.shtml

Safety

And as for the old saw argument that supplement-users are supposedly dying like flies, consider this: Over 200 million Americans take vitamin supplements. So where are the bodies? Well, there aren't any. There has not been a single death from vitamins in 27 years. http://orthomolecular.org/resources/omns/v07n05.shtml. Share that with your doctor as well. And with the news media.

(Andrew W. Saul has been an orthomolecular medical writer and lecturer for 35 years. He received the Outstanding Health Freedom Activist Award from Citizen's for Health, and is the winner of three Empire State teacher fellowships. Saul is author or coauthor of 10 books, four of which are with Abram Hoffer, M.D.)

References:

1. http://orthomolecular.org/resources/omns/v01n01.shtml

2. Saul AW. Vitamin E: A cure in search of recognition. J Orthomolecular Med, 2003. Vol 18, No 3 and 4, p 205-212. Free download at http://orthomolecular.org/library/jom/2003/pdf/2003-v18n0304-p205.pdf or html at http://www.doctoryourself.com/evitamin.htm . See also: Saul AW. Review of The vitamin E story, by Evan Shute. J Orthomolecular Med, 2002. Volume 17, Number 3, Third Quarter, p 179-181. http://www.doctoryourself.com/estory.htm

3. Klein EA, Thompson Jr, IM, Tangen CM et al. JAMA. 2011;306(14):1549-1556.

http://jama.ama-assn.org/content/306/14/1549 Also, as an example of many media spins:

http://www.webmd.com/prostate-cancer/news/20111011/vitamin-e-supplements-may-raise-prostate-cancer-risk

4. Sze Ue Luk1, Wei Ney Yap, Yung-Tuen Chiu et al. Gamma-tocotrienol as an effective agent in targeting prostate cancer stem cell-like population. International Journal of Cancer, 2011. Vol 128, No 9, p 2182-2191. http://onlinelibrary.wiley.com/doi/10.1002/ijc.25546/abstract

5. Nesaretnam K, Teoh HK, Selvaduray KR, Bruno RS, Ho E. Modulation of cell growth and apoptosis response in human prostate cancer cells supplemented with tocotrienols. Eur. J. Lipid Sci. Technol. 2008, 110, 23-31. http://onlinelibrary.wiley.com/doi/10.1002/ejlt.200700068/abstract

6. Conte C, Floridi A, Aisa C et al. Gamma-tocotrienol metabolism and antiproliferative effect in prostate cancer cells. Annals of the New York Academy of Sciences, 2004. 1031: 391-4. http://www.ncbi.nlm.nih.gov/pubmed/15753178?dopt=AbstractPlus

Free Subscription Link: http://orthomolecular.org/subscribe.html

Archives: http://orthomolecular.org/resources/omns/index.shtml

Appendix F

FOR IMMEDIATE RELEASE

Orthomolecular Medicine News Service, May 7, 2012

Dispensing with Fluoride

Editorial by Andrew W. Saul

(OMNS May 7, 2012) As a child, there was nothing I liked about going to the dental dispensary, with the possible exception of the large tropical fish aquarium in the waiting room. This was a distraction to what was coming: three hours in a vast hall containing a double line of black dental chairs and a matching double line of white-clad dental students. And that, as a six-year-old, is where I first met fluoride on a regular basis. After a free cleaning and checkup (the reason my cost-conscious parents had me go there, and the reason it literally took three hours to complete), fluoride was applied to my teeth with a swab. I remember both the smell (acrid) and the taste (astringent). I actually looked forward to the fluoride treatment, simply because it was the last thing they did to me before I was allowed to leave. Did it work? Probably not. In addition to my regular topical fluoride treatments, I lived in a city with fluoridated water and was raised on fluoridated toothpaste. And I had a mouthful of amalgam by high-school graduation.

Controversy? What Controversy?

In the late 1970s, as a young parent, I became aware of the *National Fluoridation News*, published in the still largely unknown town of Gravette, Arkansas (pop 2,200). For a very small donation, I received a boxful of back issues by return mail. In addition to this generosity, what surprised me about the *NFNews* was the high caliber of its content. Most of the non-editorial articles were well referenced and the work of well qualified scientists. This was something of a poser, for as a college biology major, I had been thoroughly schooled in the two Noble Truths of Fluoridation: 1) that fluoride in drinking water would reduce tooth decay by 60-65% and 2) that anyone who disagreed with this view was a fool. Yes, I had seen the movie *Dr. Strangelove*, and yes, I knew how to read an ADA endorsement on a toothpaste label.

Not long after this, my penchant for reading toothpaste labels paid off. There it was, printed right on the back of the tube:

"Children should only use a 'pea-sized' portion of fluoride toothpaste when they brush."

I had two toddlers, and this caught my interest. Looking into it, I learned that small children swallow a considerable quantity of toothpaste when they brush, perhaps most of it.

Anyone who has watched television at all could not have failed to see toothpaste ads. They always showed the brush loaded, with decorative overhang tips flared out on each end. When "AIM" brand toothpaste first came out, I distinctly remember toothpaste being displayed in two or even three layers on the brush. The number of children that used the product so generously, and swallowed half of it, will likely remain unknown. As for me, I immediately switched my family to toothpaste with no fluoride in it. As for toothpaste labels, they rather quickly were re-written. They now read:

"If you accidentally swallow more than used for brushing, seek professional help or contact a poison control center immediately."

But **all** children swallow more than is used for brushing. The only question is, how much? The US Centers for Disease Control states:

"Fluoride toothpaste contributes to the risk for enamel fluorosis because the swallowing reflex of children aged less than 6 years is not always well controlled, particularly among children aged less than 3 years. Children are also known to swallow toothpaste deliberately when they like its taste. A child-sized toothbrush covered with a full strip of toothpaste holds approximately 0.75-1.0 g of toothpaste, and each gram of fluoride toothpaste, as formulated in the United States, contains approximately 1.0 mg of fluoride. ***Children aged less than 6 years swallow a mean of 0.3 g of toothpaste per brushing and can inadvertently swallow as much as 0.8 g****."* [1, emphasis added]

For children age 6 and under, that is an ***average*** swallow of a third of the toothpaste they use, and a possibility of inadvertently swallowing 80% or more. There is about a milligram of fluoride in a single "serving" of toothpaste. I am calling it a "serving" because fluoride in toothpaste is regulated as if it were a food, not a drug. How is this true? Adding even less than one milligram of fluoride to a single serving of children's vitamins instantly makes them a prescription drug. It is truly odd that fluoride toothpaste remains an over-the-counter product.

Into the Schools

When my children were in grade school, the local dental college (the people who brought us the dispensary I went to as a young boy) interested our school district in a research project. Our town's public water was under local control and unfluoridated, unlike the city nearby. So the idea was to administer fluoride rinses to schoolchildren, during the school day, and then count caries. We were asked to sign a permission letter, which emphasized likely benefits and glossed over any hazards. Remembering what youngsters did with sweet toothpaste, I made a guess that they'd swallow a saccharin-laced rinse about as well. We chose to not sign. But I did check the box to receive results of the study. It ultimately came in the form of a letter, saying that the results were disappointingly inconclusive: no evidence that fluoride rinses helped our unfluoridated-water-drinking community. I am unaware that the study was published.

That is not especially surprising. Shutting out access to balanced scientific discussion of fluoridation is alive and well...and taxpayer supported. Negative fluoride studies and reviews are hardly abundant on PubMed/Medline. One does not need to be a conspiracy theorist to observe that the US National Library of Medicine refuses to index the journal *Fluoride*. [2] Censorship is conspicuously aberrant behavior for any public library.

No Discussion

About 15 years ago, our town's public water supply was annexed by the nearby metropolis. Aside from a rate increase, the only other, barely detectable change to our bill was a one-time typed legend at the bottom of it that fluoride has now been added to the water. There had been no vote, and there had not even been any discussion. Communities coast-to-coast know that this is not at all uncommon. Four glasses of fluoridated tap water contain about as much fluoride as a prescription dose does. Not only is fluoridated water nonprescription, it is even more certain to be swallowed than toothpaste. Being over 6 years of age means better control over swallowing reflexes, thus limiting ingestion of fluoride from toothpaste. There is no such accommodation for drinking water.

Evidence-based medicine requires evidence before medicating. Fluoridation of water is not evidence-based. It has not been tested in well-controlled studies. Fluoridation of public water is a default medication, since you have to deliberately avoid it if you do not want to take it. A person's daily intake of fluoride simply from drinking an average quantity of fluoridated tap water, fluoridated bottled water, and beverages produced or prepared with fluoridated water can easily exceed the threshold for what your druggist would rightly demand a prescription for. Fluoride in toothpaste and mouth rinses also is medication. It may be intended as topical, but the reality is different. No matter how it may be applied in their mouths, young children are going to swallow it. Indeed, most of the public and the dental profession already have.

References:

1. Fluoride Recommendations Work Group. Recommendations for using fluoride to prevent and control dental caries in the United States. CDC Recommendations and Reports 2001;50(RR14):1-42. http://www.cdc.gov/mmwr/preview/mmwrhtml/rr5014a1.htm

2. http://www.orthomolecular.org/resources/omns/v06n05.shtml If you want access to what the US taxpayer-funded National Library of Medicine refuses to index, you may read over 40 years' of articles from the journal Fluoride, free of charge, at http://www.fluorideresearch.org/ Scroll down to "Archives and Indexes,1968-2011."

Comment by Albert W. Burgstahler, PhD: Support for these views and conclusions is found in a recent review in *Critical Public Health* (2011:1-19) titled "Slaying sacred cows: is it time to pull the plug on water fluoridation?" by Stephen Peckham of the Department of Health Services Research and Policy, London School of Hygiene and Tropical Medicine. In his article, Peckham concludes that evidence for the effectiveness and safety of water fluoridation is seriously defective and not in agreement with findings of a growing body of current and previously overlooked research. For an abstract of this report, scroll down at: http://www.fluorideresearch.org/444/files/FJ2011_v44_n4_p260-261_sfs.pdf

This revised article originally appeared in Fluoride 2011, 44(4)188-190. It is reprinted with kind permission of the International Society for Fluoride Research Inc. www.fluorideresearch.org or www.fluorideresearch.com. Editorial Office: 727 Brighton Road, Ocean View, Dunedin 9035, New Zealand.

Free Subscription Link: http://orthomolecular.org/subscribe.html

Archives: http://orthomolecular.org/resources/omns/index.shtml

Appendix G.1

FOR IMMEDIATE RELEASE

Orthomolecular Medicine News Service, January 17, 2012

Supplements: The Real Story

Natural or Synthetic? Foods or Tablets?

(OMNS, Jan 17, 2012) It's a nutritional "Catch 22": The public is told, confusingly: *"Vitamins are good, but vitamin supplements are not. Only vitamins from food will help you. So just eat a good diet. Do not take supplements! But by the way, there is no difference between natural and synthetic vitamins."*

Wait a minute. What's the real story here?

A recent health study reported that the risk of heart failure decreased with increasing blood levels of vitamin C [1]. The benefit of vitamin C (ascorbate) was highly significant. Persons with the lowest plasma levels of ascorbate had the highest risk of heart failure, and ***persons with the highest levels of vitamin C had the lowest risk of heart failure.*** This finding confirms the knowledge derived over the last 50 years that vitamin C is a major essential factor in cardiovascular health [2,3]. The study raises several important questions about diet and vitamin supplements.

Was it Food or Supplements?

The report discussed vitamin C as if it were simply an indicator of how many fruits and vegetables were consumed by the participants. Yet, ironically, the study's results show little improvement in the risk for heart failure from consuming fruits and vegetables. This implies that the real factor in reducing the risk was indeed the amount of vitamin C consumed. Moreover, the study appears to utterly ignore the widespread use of vitamin C supplements to improve cardiovascular health. In fact, out of four quartile groups, the quartile ***with the highest plasma vitamin C had six to ten times the rate of vitamin C supplementation*** of the lowest quartile, but this fact was not emphasized. This type of selective attention to food sources of vitamin C, while dismissing supplements as an important source, appears to be an attempt to marginalize the importance of vitamin supplements.

Many medical and nutritional reports have maintained that there is little difference between natural and synthetic vitamins. This is known to be true for some essential nutrients. The ascorbate found in widely available vitamin C tablets is identical to the ascorbate found in fruits and vegetables [3]. Linus Pauling emphasized this fact, and explained how ordinary vitamin C, inexpensively manufactured from glucose, could improve health in many important ways [4]. Indeed, the above-mentioned study specifically measured the plasma level of ascorbate, which was shown to be an important factor associated with lower risk of heart failure [1, 2]. The study did not measure blood plasma levels of the components of fruits and vegetables. It measured vitamin C.

A known rationale for this dramatic finding is that vitamin C helps to prevent inflammation in the arteries by several mechanisms. It is a necessary co-factor for the synthesis of collagen, which is a major component of arteries. Vitamin C is also an important antioxidant throughout the body that can help to recycle other antioxidants like vitamin E and glutathione in the artery walls [2,3]. This was underscored by a report that ***high plasma levels of vitamin C are associated with a 50% reduction in risk for stroke*** [5].

Yes, Synthetic Vitamin C is Clinically Effective

We can almost hear "Unsubscribe" links being clicked as we state it, but here it is: synthetic vitamin C works, in real people with real illnesses. Ascorbate's efficacy has little direct relation to food intake. A dramatic case of this was a dairy farmer in New Zealand who was on life support with lung whiteout, kidney failure, leukemia and swine flu. He was given 100,000 mg of vitamin C daily and his life was saved. We have nothing against oranges or other vitamin C-containing foods. Fruits and vegetables are good for you for many, many reasons. However, you'll need to get out your calculator to help you figure out how many oranges it would take to get that much, and then also figure how to get a sick person to eat them all.

It is established that liver function improves with vitamin C supplementation, and it is equally well known that adequate levels of vitamin C are essential for the proper functioning of the immune system. Vitamin C improves the ability of the white blood cells to fight bacteria and viruses. OMNS has more articles expanding on this topic, available for free access at http://orthomolecular.org/resources/omns/index.shtml.

Deficiency of vitamin C is very common. According to US Department of Agriculture (USDA) data, [7] ***nearly half of Americans do not get even the US RDA of vitamin C***, which is a mere 90 mg.

Synthetic Vitamin E is Less Effective

For some other nutrients, there is a significant difference in efficacy between synthetic and natural forms. Vitamin E is a crucial anti-oxidant, but also has other functions in the body, not all well understood. It comprises eight different biochemical forms, alpha-, beta-, delta- and gamma tocopherols, and alpha-, beta-, delta-, and gamma-tocotrienols. All of these forms of vitamin E are important for the body. Current knowledge about the function of vitamin E is rapidly expanding, and each of the eight forms of natural vitamin E is thought to have a slightly different function in the body. For example, gamma-tocotrienol actually kills prostate cancer stem cells better than chemotherapy does. (http://orthomolecular.org/resources/omns/v07n11.shtml)

Synthetic vitamin E is widely available and inexpensive. It is "DL-alpha-tocopherol." Yes, it has the same antioxidant properties in test tube experiments as does the natural "D-alpha-tocopherol" form. However, the DL- form has only 50% of the biological efficacy, because the body utilizes only the natural D isomer, which comprises half of the synthetic mix [8]. Therefore, studies utilizing DL-alpha-tocopherol that do not take this fact into account are starting with an already-halved dose that will naturally lead to a reduction in the observed efficacy.

Then there are the esterified forms of vitamin E such as acetate or succinate. These esterified forms, either natural or synthetic, have a greater shelf life because the ester protects the vitamin E from being oxidized and neutralized. When acid in the stomach cleaves the acetate or succinate component from the original natural vitamin E molecule, the gut can then absorb a good fraction and the body receives its antioxidant benefit. But when esterified vitamin E acetate is applied to the skin to prevent inflammation, it is ineffective because there is no acid present to remove the acetate ester.

Based on USDA data [9] an astonishing ***90% of Americans do not get the RDA of vitamin E***, which is, believe it or not, under 23 IU (15mg) per day.

Magnesium Deficiency is Widespread

Magnesium is another example. ***Over two-thirds of the population do not get the RDA of magnesium.***[10] Deficiency can cause a wide variety of symptoms, including osteoporosis, high blood pressure, heart disease, asthma, depression, and diabetes. Magnesium can be purchased in many forms. The most widely available form is magnesium oxide, which is not very effective because it is only about 5% absorbed [11]. Magnesium oxide supplements are popular because the pills are smaller—they contain more magnesium, but won't help most people. Better forms of magnesium are magnesium citrate, magnesium malate, and the best absorbed is magnesium chloride. It's always good to consult your doctor to determine your ideal intake. Testing may reveal unexpected deficiency. [12]

Well, Which? Natural or Synthetic?

While the natural form of vitamin E (mixed natural tocopherols and tocotrienols) is at least twice as effective as the synthetic form, this is not true of vitamin C. The ascorbate that the body gets from fruits and vegetables is the same as the ascorbate in vitamin C tablets. On first thought, this may sound confusing, because there are many so-called "natural" forms of vitamin C widely available. But ***virtually every study that demonstrated that supplemental vitamin C fights illness used plain, cheap, synthetic ascorbic acid.*** Other forms of ascorbate, for instance, the sodium or magnesium salt of ascorbic acid, are digested slightly differently by the gut, but once the ascorbate molecule is absorbed from these forms, it has identical efficacy. The advantage of these ascorbate salts is that they are non-acidic and can be ingested or topically applied to any part of the body without concern about irritation from acidity.

Further, it is known that essential nutrients are symbiotic, that is, they are more effective when taken as a group in proper doses. For example, vitamin E is more effective when taken along with vitamin C and selenium, because each of these essential nutrients can improve the efficacy of the others. Similarly, the B vitamins are more effective when taken together. Readers with dosage questions will want to consult their healthcare provider, and also look at freely available information archived at http://orthomolecular.org/resources/omns/index.shtml.

Food Factors

Natural food factors are also important. Bioflavonoids and other vitamin C-friendly components in fresh fruits and vegetables (sometimes called "vitamin C complex") do indeed have health benefits. These natural components are easily obtained from a healthy, unprocessed whole foods diet. However, eating even a very good diet does not supply nearly enough vitamin C to be effective against illness. A really good diet might provide several hundred milligrams of vitamin C daily. An extreme raw food diet might provide two or three thousand milligrams of vitamin C, but this is not practical for most people. Supplementation, with a good diet, is.

The principle that "natural" vitamins are better than synthetic vitamins is a widely quoted justification for actually avoiding vitamin supplements. The argument goes, because vitamins and minerals are available from food in their natural form, that somehow one might suppose that we are best off by ignoring supplements. Apparently this is what the authors of the above-mentioned study had in mind, because the report hardly mentions vitamin supplements.

Conclusion

In the real world of today's processed food, most of us don't get all the nutrients we need in adequate doses. *Most people are deficient in* ***several*** *of the essential nutrients.* These deficiencies are responsible for much suffering, including heart disease, cancer, premature aging, dementia, diabetes, and other diseases such as eye disease, multiple sclerosis and asthma. The above-mentioned study showing the efficacy of vitamin C in reducing heart failure is but one of the many studies showing the value of vitamins. Others are discussed and available at http://orthomolecular.org/resources/omns/index.shtml .

For vitamin E, the natural form, taken in adequate doses along with a nutritious diet, is the best medicine. However, for most vitamins, including vitamin C, the manufactured form is identical to the natural one. Both are biologically active and both work clinically. It all comes down to dose. Supplements enable optimum intake; foods alone do not.

Don't be fooled: nutrient deficiency is the rule, not the exception. That's why we need supplements. When ill, we need them even more.

References:

1. Pfister R, Sharp SJ, Luben R, Wareham NJ, Khaw KT. (2011) Plasma vitamin C predicts incident heart failure in men and women in European Prospective Investigation into Cancer and Nutrition-Norfolk prospective study. Am Heart J. 162:246-253. See also: http://orthomolecular.org/resources/omns/v07n14.shtml

2. Levy TE (2006) Stop America's #1 Killer: Reversible Vitamin Deficiency Found to be Origin of All Coronary Heart Disease. ISBN-13: 9780977952007

3. Hickey S, Saul AW (2008) Vitamin C: The Real Story, the Remarkable and Controversial Healing Factor. Basic Health Publications, ISBN-13: 978-1591202233

4. Pauling L. (2006) How to Live Longer And Feel Better. Oregon State University Press, Corvallis, OR. ISBN-13: 9780870710964

5. Kurl S, Tuomainen TP, Laukkanen JA, Nyyssönen K, Lakka T, Sivenius J, Salonen JT. (2002) Plasma vitamin C modifies the association between hypertension and risk of stroke. Stroke. 33:1568-1573

7. Free, full text paper at http://www.ncbi.nlm.nih.gov/pmc/articles/PMC1405127/pdf/amjph00225-0021.pdf

8. Papas A. (1999) The Vitamin E Factor: The miraculous antioxidant for the prevention and treatment of heart disease, cancer, and aging. HarperCollins, NY. ISBN-13: 9780060984434

9. http://lpi.oregonstate.edu/infocenter/vitamins/vitaminE/ ; scroll down to "Deficiency."

10. Free, full text paper at http://www.jacn.org/content/24/3/166.full.pdf+html (or http://www.jacn.org/content/24/3/166.long)

11. Dean, C. (2007) The Magnesium Miracle. Ballantine Books, ISBN-13: 9780345494580

12. http://www.doctoryourself.com/epilepsy.html

Free Subscription Link: http://orthomolecular.org/subscribe.html

Archives: http://orthomolecular.org/resources/omns/index.shtml

Appendix G.2

FOR IMMEDIATE RELEASE

Orthomolecular Medicine News Service, December 28, 2011

No Deaths from Vitamins

America's Largest Database Confirms Supplement Safety

(OMNS, Dec 28, 2011) There was not even one death caused by a vitamin supplement in 2010, according to the most recent information collected by the U.S. National Poison Data System.

The new 203-page annual report of the American Association of Poison Control Centers, published online at http://www.aapcc.org/dnn/Portals/0/2010%20NPDS%20Annual%20Report.pdf, shows zero deaths from multiple vitamins; zero deaths from any of the B vitamins; zero deaths from vitamins A, C, D, or E; and zero deaths from any other vitamin.

Additionally, there were no deaths whatsoever from any amino acid or dietary mineral supplement.

Three people died from non-supplement mineral poisoning: two from medical use of sodium and one from non-supplemental iron. On page 131, the AAPCC report specifically indicates that the iron fatality was not from a nutritional supplement.

Fifty-seven poison centers provide coast-to-coast data for the National Poison Data System, "one of the few real-time national surveillance systems in existence, providing a model public health surveillance system for all types of exposures, public health event identification, resilience response and situational awareness tracking."

Well over half of the U.S. population takes daily nutritional supplements. Even if each of those people took only one single tablet daily, that makes 165,000,000 individual doses per day, for a total of over 60 billion doses annually. Since many persons take far more than just one single vitamin or mineral tablet, actual consumption is considerably higher, and the safety of nutritional supplements is all the more remarkable.

Over 60 billion doses of vitamin and mineral supplements per year in the USA, and not a single fatality. Not one.

If vitamin and mineral supplements are allegedly so "dangerous," as the FDA and news media so often claim, then ***where are the bodies?***

Reference:

Bronstein AC, Spyker DA, Cantilena LR Jr, Green JL, Rumack BH, Dart RC. 2010 Annual Report of the American Association of Poison Control Centers' National Poison Data System (NPDS): 28th Annual Report. The full text article is available for free download at http://www.aapcc.org/dnn/Portals/0/2010%20NPDS%20Annual%20Report.pdf

The data mentioned above are found in Table 22B. Mineral data on page 131; vitamin data on pages 137-139.

Free Subscription Link: http://orthomolecular.org/subscribe.html

Archives: http://orthomolecular.org/resources/omns/index.shtml

Appendix G.3

FOR IMMEDIATE RELEASE

Orthomolecular Medicine News Service, January 23, 2012

The War Against Nutritional Medicine

Why We Love Our Critics

by Andrew W. Saul, OMNS Editor

(OMNS, Jan 23, 2012) When physicians criticized Linus Pauling for advocating vitamin C, Dr. Pauling wrote a book that became an all-time nutritional bestseller: *Vitamin C and the Common Cold.* (1) It won the Phi Beta Kappa Award in Science. Then, after he and colleagues demonstrated that vitamin C fights cancer, he was attacked again. When medical orthodoxy prevented him from publishing timely rebuttals in their pharma-funded journals, Pauling wrote more books. (2,3) When critics go after the Gerson nutritional therapy, Charlotte Gerson writes another book. (4) She will turn 90 on March 24. The more efforts to silence, the more education gets out.

When psychiatric journals refused to publish Abram Hoffer's controlled studies showing that niacin cured many forms of mental illness, Dr. Hoffer started his own *Journal of Orthomolecular Medicine.* (5) When scientific journals refused to publish studies questioning water fluoridation, the journal *Fluoride* was started to get the research in print. (6) Someday, you might actually be able to find these journals at the US National Library of Medicine/Medline. But don't hold your breath. NLM, your taxpayer-supported "largest medical library on earth," censors your access to journals it does not like. (7) Worldwide, as well as in the United States of America, most people feel that such behavior from a public library is reprehensible. If you are among these who do, you can write to NLM's

Medline boss and tell him so. (8) They will not let you write to committee members, who make their decisions in closed meetings. (9)

Every time pharmaphilic opponents of nutritional medicine try to monopolize the news media, the Orthomolecular Medicine News service publishes another press release or two, directly to the public. OMNS articles are all over the internet, and there have been 120 different releases, all free of charge and without advertising. http://orthomolecular.org/resources/omns/ Thank you for your continued interest and support.

Not everyone likes this newsfeed. Most of the media ignore it. Not surprising. Perhaps they think that no one is searching the internet for a second opinion, and that people only read and believe what they, the major magazines and newspapers, select as fit to print. Maybe the TV networks have forgotten about YouTube, and websites where there is a growing presence of free-access orthomolecular video. (10)

And as for Wikipedia, if you want to read what cliques of amateurs have need to say about subjects that do or do not fit their belief systems, be our guest. I taught for the State University of New York for nine years, and I never met a single faculty member that would pay the slightest heed to a Wikipedia reference. They know better. You know better. That is why OMNS goes directly to academics, researchers, and physicians for information and commentary. Many years ago, my father taught me that when you want to know, "Go to the organ grinder, not the monkey."

As you read this, the medical monopoly is melting like an iceberg in the Panama Canal. Nutritional medicine is catching on worldwide. Original case reports and research papers of Dr. Max Gerson are, this minute, being translated from German into English for the first time ever. They will be published for free access online this year. No longer will cancer organizations get away with rhetoric such as, "If the Gerson approach worked, there would be evidence that demonstrates it." Well, it does, and there is. If your doctor does not know this, teach him or her to click a mouse button.

We love piquing the medical industry. We are grateful for our critics. We love it when they respond, because we just go ahead and issue yet another OMNS release showing how nutritional therapy is proven safe and effective. When they don't respond, we will keep provoking them until they do. For example, let them explain these:

- A Harvard study showed a *27% decrease in deaths among AIDS patients taking vitamin supplements.* (11)
- There has never been a single death from a vitamin. That's right: zero. (12)
- Women who take two aspirin tablets per day have an 86 percent greater risk of pancreatic cancer. (13)
- Milligram for milligram, vitamin supplementation is cheaper than trying to get vitamins from food. (14)

Here is the latest thorn in Big Pharma's paw. Starting Feb 1, the *Orthomolecular Medicine News Service* will be available in Japanese, thanks to the Japanese College of Intravenous Therapy, the Japanese Society of Orthomolecular Medicine, and other progressive medical organizations.

We are not going to rest with that. If you are multilingual and interested in volunteering to translate OMNS releases into other languages, please write in and let us know. You can pick the release http://orthomolecular.org/resources/omns/ and you can pick the language.

Vitamin and nutrient therapy is safer and more effective than drug therapy. Let's get this message out to every person, everywhere, in every language.

References:

1. Pauling L. (1970) Vitamin C, the Common Cold, and the Flu. San Francisco: W. H. Freeman. Revised edition, 1976.

2. Cameron E, Pauling L. (1979) Cancer and Vitamin C. Linus Pauling Institute of Science and Medicine, Menlo Park, CA. Warner Books, New York 1981; Revised edition, 1993, Philadelphia: Camino Books.

3. Pauling L. (1986) How to Live Longer and Feel Better. New York: W. H. Freeman. Revised and updated edition, 2006, Corvallis, OR:

Oregon State University Press. Reviewed at http://www.doctoryourself.com/livelonger.html

4. Gerson C. (2011) Defeating Arthritis, Bone and Joint Diseases. Carmel, CA: Gerson Health Media. Also: (2010) Defeating Obesity, Diabetes and High Blood Pressure: The Metabolic Syndrome. Carmel, CA: Gerson Health Media. And: (2007) Healing the Gerson Way: Defeating Cancer and Other Chronic Diseases. Totality Books. Reviewed at http://orthomolecular.org/library/jom/2007/pdf/2007-v22n04-p217.pdf Also: (2001) Gerson C, Walker, M. The Gerson Therapy. NY: Kensington Publishing.

5. Free access to archive at http://orthomolecular.org/library/jom/

6. Free access to archive at http://www.fluorideresearch.org/

7. http://orthomolecular.org/resources/omns/v06n03.shtml and http://orthomolecular.org/resources/omns/v06n07.shtml

8. Sheldon Kotzin, Executive Editor, MEDLINE, National Library of Medicine, Bethesda, Maryland kotzins@mail.nlm.nih.gov This email was verified Jan 19. 2012.

9. http://www.doctoryourself.com/medline.html , scroll about halfway down the page.

10. Intravenous vitamin C instructional videos for doctors: http://orthomolecular.org/resources/omns/v07n03.shtml

11. Fawzi WW, Msamanga GI, Spiegelman D, Wei R, Kapiga S, Villamor E, Mwakagile D, Mugusi F, Hertzmark E, Essex M, Hunter DJ. A Randomized Trial of Multivitamin Supplements and HIV Disease Progression and Mortality. N Engl J Med. 2004 Jul 1;351(1):23-32. Free full text article at http://www.nejm.org/doi/pdf/10.1056/NEJMoa040541

12. Most recent year: http://orthomolecular.org/resources/omns/v07n16.shtml Previous 27 years: http://orthomolecular.org/resources/omns/v07n05.shtml

13. http://orthomolecular.org/resources/omns/v07n12.shtml

14. A single large orange costs at least 50 cents and may easily cost one dollar. It provides less than 100 milligrams (mg) of vitamin C. A bottle of 100 tablets of ascorbic acid vitamin C, 500 mg each, costs

about five dollars. The supplement gives you 10,000 mg per dollar. In terms of vitamin C, the supplement is 50 to 100 times cheaper, costing about one or two cents for the amount of vitamin C in an orange.

Free Subscription Link: http://orthomolecular.org/subscribe.html

Archives: http://orthomolecular.org/resources/omns/index.shtml

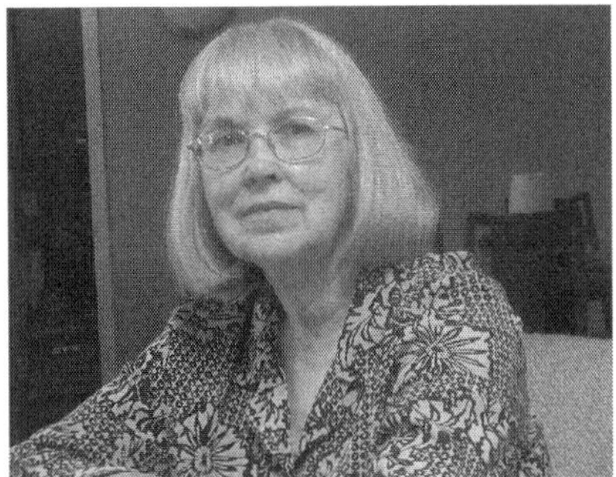

About the Author

Carole Ramke is the proprietor of Wildwood Eco-Farm in the Piney Woods of East Texas. She and her husband have a small flock of laying hens and their property is shared with deer, bobcats, coyotes, foxes and various smaller critters.

Carole is a local food proponent and hosts monthly meetings of Northeast Texas Organic Gardeners. In addition to researching and gardening, she enjoys spending time with her children and grandchildren.

www.howtostopcolds.com

About the Cover Artist

Don Auderer is a self-taught photographer who began to pursue photography with a passion after his retirement. Photographic prints are made using the latest digital techniques and include archival pigment inks and papers. He has won numerous awards in the Texas Bank and Trust Photography Contest including "best of show" in 2007. His work has been exhibited in Tyler and Austin. He was also one of the artists featured in the East Texas Regional Artist Show at the Longview Museum of Fine Art in July of 2012.

Artist's Statement: I use my camera as a painter would use a sketchpad to capture quickly a visual idea. Then, I take the image to my digital darkroom, refining it and exploring the possibilities of how to present it to the viewer. Some work is "as shot" straight from the camera while other work may include extensive post-processing. I prefer to work in black and white because it offers a great deal of creative freedom along every step of the process from exposure to printing. In terms of pure visual enjoyment, black and white provides the beauty of tonal values that so richly express the play of light and shadow – shades of grey and deep blacks and bright whites. Photography challenges me to "see" as well as look, to turn the mundane into art, and to find new ways of presenting the world around me.

www.pbase.com/donauderer